MIDWI
A JOURNEY

by
Peggy Vincent, RN, CNM.

Author of *Baby Catcher: Chronicles of a Modern Midwife*
Scribner, Simon & Schuster 2002
and
Midwife: A Calling
Ant Press 2015

BOOK II
MEMOIRS OF AN URBAN MIDWIFE

Also available in Large Print and eBook editions.

Contents

To all the women having their first babies at home
not knowing how long it will last
not knowing what it will feel like
not knowing, really, how hard it can be

yet still they trust
and triumph

Some couples whose stories appear in these pages have generously given permission for their real names to be used. In those cases, I have stayed as true to actual events as our shared memories permit.

For the rest, pseudonyms are used for the sake of privacy.

In addition, some characters are composites. Dates, locations, and personal details may have been altered for the purpose of narrative flow.

If errors are found, they are solely mine.

Critical Decision

I felt my life had been blessed.

Except for the catastrophic end to my first pregnancy, including the loss of an ovary, a Fallopian tube, and a piece of omentum (sort of a fatty apron that protects the abdominal organs), everything I'd dreamed of, planned for, and worked toward in my life had come to fruition. I had very little experience with failure or disappointment.

After years as a delivery room nurse and two years of managing the hospital's alternative birth center, I had reached a crossroads. I had some critical decisions to make.

I had a pretty cushy deal at the hospital. I was one of the few remaining day shift nurses whose contract stipulated full benefits not only for me but also for my family, yet required me to put in only three eight-hour shifts a week. I had friends as colleagues, and I loved my job. I was confident, I knew I was good at what I did, and I had plenty of time off to be with my family.

But I had sneaked a peek into the future. I began to feel frustration when an obstetrician appeared in the birth center and asserted his (or her) personality or objectives, disrupting the sweet and careful balance the laboring couple and I had created. One memorable afternoon, soft classical music played in the dimly lit birthing room where the laboring mom crooned quietly to herself during contractions. Her partner cradled her in his strong arms and whispered into her ear while I stroked her hair and murmured encouragement now and then. Nothing more was needed.

Suddenly the door banged open, the overhead lights flared on, and the doctor's loud voice interrupted the tranquility we'd all worked so hard to establish.

"Okay, what's taking so long here? Let me check you and see if we can get this show on the road."

Too often I was forced to stand by and watch the interruption of an entirely normal labor process by a well-intentioned but sorely out-of-touch doctor who really didn't appear to understand the concept of normal, natural birth.

I sometimes wondered if any of the obstetricians had seen a truly natural birth. They certainly hadn't gone through years and years of schooling to "do nothing," so just sitting on their hands and watching didn't exactly come easily to them.

As similar scenarios happened again and again, I began to feel that, if I stayed on as a staff nurse and manager of the birthing center, I was in danger of becoming jaded, frustrated, or complicit…and none of those alternatives were acceptable.

At the same time, several of the Higher Ups in the administration were putting not-so-subtle pressure on me to jump ship, abandon the ranks of my coworkers, and join the administrative staff. They didn't realize it, but I felt this would be a big mistake. They'd seen only my organizational skills in writing up the protocols for the birth center and my tenacity in shepherding the entire concept through endless committees and, finally, into its very existence. They saw me as Someone Who Got Things Done.

What they didn't recognize is what a terrible committee member I really am. I'm a believer in the axiom that "A camel is a horse designed by a committee," and as such, I have a short fuse when it comes to compromise. To be a good administrator, one needs to play well with others, and that's never really been one of my better skills.

Another option, the one so many of my friends saw as the obvious choice, was to become a midwife. It's the path I eventually followed, of course, but I had to consider what I would be losing: job security, medical coverage for the whole family, vacation time, paid holidays, sick pay, a pension plan, regular hours…my whole way of life.

It was a sacrifice in many ways, but a relief in so many others. In spite of the hurdles looming ahead, I would have continued satisfaction in doing my job: caring for pregnant women and their families, getting to know them, helping them reach their individual goals, offering my knowledge and skills and midwifery arts to choreograph with them a birth as close to their dreams as possible.

So the die was cast. In January of 1980, I began midwifery school at San Francisco General Hospital through the auspices of the University of California at San Francisco.

* * *

At the beginning of midwifery school, I assumed I would graduate and have a hospital-based practice. I assumed that, during my training, somehow the wheels would be set in place for midwives to apply for privileges at Alta Bates Hospital. I assumed the well-respected hospital where I'd been a delivery room nurse for the past decade would give me delivery privileges and that I'd find an obstetrician willing, even eager, to provide backup.

I assumed, as I told myself over and over, This Will Work Out.

There were twelve of us midwife students. We came from divergent backgrounds with varying skills and experience, but we all shared a common goal: to practice the Art of Midwifery, not the science of obstetrics.

Some wanted to care for underserved women in county hospitals or rural areas. Some intended to resume their previous association with a physician but now as a midwife instead of as a nurse practitioner. Some planned to return to their old home birth practices, but now legal and with the ability to purchase malpractice insurance.

I assumed I would apply for and obtain hospital privileges and be able to manage my laboring clients and catch their babies, and if complications arose, doctors would be available to back me up. Sympatico obstetricians. Obstetricians who wanted the same thing I did: for women to have a choice as to their care provider.

Call me naïve.

I was wrong...and about four months before I graduated from midwifery school, I was forced to give serious thought to what on earth I was actually going to do with this degree I was about to receive.

Prior to beginning midwifery school, I'd been on a trajectory. Beginning as an OB staff nurse, I'd progressed to becoming a charge nurse and moved on to become the founder of the birth center at Alta Bates. I had many close friends among the nurses, and I got along well with the majority of the obstetricians. I felt they trusted and respected me, and I believed the majority of them liked me. I think I figured I would just slide more or less effortlessly into practicing midwifery at the hospital where I'd been a nurse.

In retrospect, I imagine the doctors were aware of my intentions. And I suspect that as soon as I left for midwifery school, they closed ranks. To be fair, there were several, perhaps as many as ten, who were favorably disposed to at least the "idea" of a nurse-midwife in a collegial relationship with them. But most were threatened by the possibility.

Think about it.

Midwives focus their skills on normal and healthy women experiencing uncomplicated pregnancies. To obstetricians, these women are the bread and butter of their practice. They charged big bucks to care for such women. And what did those fees include?

- An initial prenatal visit lasting half an hour
- About ten follow-up visits lasting perhaps ten minutes each
- Two or three quick visits during labor "to evaluate progress"
- Half an hour for attending the delivery itself, sometimes far less.

That adds up to less than maybe three hours of the doctor's time.

Pretty good money for bread and butter. Money they were reluctant to share.

But of course they couldn't use that fact as a legitimate objection. It would make them appear churlish and greedy. So they conjured up other reasons, the primary one being their declaration that midwives aren't trained to handle complications.

However, midwives all over the world, particularly in remote and rural areas – and especially in Third World countries – handle complications in the total absence of physicians. And midwives in large county hospitals or HMOs manage complications of varying degrees of severity according to their practice guidelines.

Here's the real picture. If midwives are employed by a physician group or a hospital group, then the obstetricians are generally delighted to have them on staff beside them. Why?

Money.

Money, time, and convenience.

The midwives care for the laboring women, allowing the doctors to go home, eat with their families, sleep, go on with their lives or office hours or surgeries, confident they won't have to make an appearance unless there is a problem.

Midwives will accept night and holiday shifts.

Midwives are on salary.

These midwives don't threaten physicians, because the midwives are their employees…and they make the doctors' jobs and lives oh, so much easier.

But let that same midwife try to set up a private practice, billing insurance companies independently and collecting full fees for services rendered – in essence, running her own business – and resistance rises and doors slam shut.

As I neared the end of midwifery school, I saw the proverbial writing on the wall and understood that I faced some insurmountable obstacles. When she heard I had hoped to apply for privileges at Alta Bates, the director of our program commented that I was "sucking on a dry tit" if I thought it would happen by my graduation at the end of December 1980…if ever.

And I was sure she was right.

So. What was Plan B?

I was tired of following doctors' orders. I wanted freedom, independence, and as much autonomy as possible. Other than accepting a position as a midwife at the county hospital on a team supervised by obstetricians, a role I wasn't interested in, there were really no options open to me other than home birth.

So I stepped into the unknown.

I Deserve a Break Today

In the early Seventies, when a doctor arrived too late for a birth, we were obligated to call the physician working in the Emergency Room. All the doctors on the staff took turns signing on for an occasional shift, because this was an era before Trauma was a separate area in which doctors could specialize.

This served our OB patients poorly, as sometimes the physician who answered our call might be an ear, nose, and throat specialist, or a thoracic surgeon who hadn't been within twenty feet of a laboring woman since medical school. Such doctors didn't feel confident in the delivery room, and we OB nurses agreed with their self-assessment. It didn't take long before we just stopped calling them and began handling the births ourselves. After all, babies that come too fast for the obstetrician to make it in time are usually quick and easy catches, rarely requiring more than a calm presence and a modicum of experience. Any nurse who has worked a couple of years with birthing women has probably caught a few babies on her own.

As part of fulfilling the requirements for graduation, each of us student midwives had to catch twenty babies under the direct supervision of a licensed midwife or obstetrician. As a delivery room nurse with years of experience, I'd already caught well over a hundred babies at the hospital.

When it became public knowledge that I was heading for midwifery school, a couple of doctors who were supportive, encouraged me to go ahead and conduct the delivery of a woman I'd been caring for in labor, with the woman's permission, of course. "Just so you have as much experience as possible before you strike out on your own," as Dr. Bill Stallone said to me one afternoon.

I recall a situation in the birth center in which the woman was on her hands and knees, pushing. When Bill came into the room, he looked at her, donned a scrub gown and gloves, and then watched her for a while longer.

"Is she planning on staying that way?" he asked. He was very quiet, very polite. He didn't assert himself into the situation or make demands. It was just a simple question.

"Kind of looks like it," I said.

"I've never done a birth that way," he said.

"Mmm…"

"Have you?"

"Yeah, a couple. You just kind of do everything upside-down."

"Well, how about you do this one while I watch?"

So I did.

And so did he. He watched. He just stood there with his gloved hands folded at his waist, and he watched the baby slide out looking straight up at the ceiling.

As I passed the baby between her mother's legs and into her arms, Bill just said, "Huh. Okay, I could do that, I guess." He took a quick peek to be sure no suturing was needed, said, "Good job, ma'am. Lovely baby," and he walked out.

Now, we could do with more of that kind of obstetrician. And less of the kind that too frequently seem to want to make themselves the center of attention, the hero riding in on a white horse to "save" a situation that never needed saving in the first place.

Thus, I entered the last few months of our year's training with a fair number of baby catches already under my belt. One of my classmates, however, had had no delivery experience whatsoever, so the director asked me if I would "give some of my births to her." I agreed, of course, but then, oddly, babies didn't seem to want to come into the world on my shifts, and it began to look as though I would be short on my own numbers.

Then my phone started ringing, and suddenly I had a queue of several women wanting home births whose due dates were well before the end of the year. The only snag was that these births had to be supervised in order to count toward the twenty required for graduation.

Out of nothing more than the goodness of her heart and a generous willingness to mentor new midwives following in her footsteps, Carole Hagin, a midwife of many years experience with seven children of her own (and a very cooperative husband) agreed to show up at those births. They would count toward my numbers, provided everything went smoothly and they could all give birth at home.

But what if one of these women actually did require a transfer to the hospital? Three had already had babies, and chances were good they'd be able to give birth at home. But two of them were first-timers. I knew from years of experience that true life-and-death emergencies in obstetrics are rare, but a first time mom cursed with a grueling, nasty labor spanning two or three days will probably end up at the hospital...just because of sheer exhaustion, not because there is any real emergency. It would not be a home birth, and I would not be catching the baby, but I had to somehow arrange for such an event, just in case.

So, in addition to Carole's agreement to be present for home births, I had to find an obstetrician who would agree to back me up for a potential hospital transfer. Bill Stallone agreed immediately to my tentative request, and to my surprise, he offered to continue that backup support after my graduation. I wouldn't be able to continue managing the care of my clients, nor would I officially be allowed to deliver them at the hospital, but my pregnant clients would receive excellent care by a compassionate doctor whose heart and hands were mostly those of a midwife.

* * *

It was late in August when I received a phone call from Chana, who was to become my first private client. She requested that I attend the birth of her first baby at home.

I was nonplussed.

"Uh...hi. But...wait. How did you hear about me? I haven't even finished midwifery school yet."

"I called Alta Bates and asked the woman who answered the phone if there were any midwives on the staff. She said, 'No. Well...not yet, anyway,' and she gave me your phone number."

"We should talk," I said, and I took down a few notes on what would become my first private client's chart. Then I asked, "I'm curious about your reason for coming to me so late in your pregnancy."

"It's taken me this long to admit to myself that I don't really like my obstetrician. And I don't trust him. He says he won't do anything to me as long as everything is normal, but I just get the feeling his definition of normal might not be the same as mine. I've read that *Spiritual Midwifery* book and figured, well, why not have a home birth with a midwife? My two sisters had pretty normal, quick births with

15

their first babies, so why should it be any different for me?"

Actually, Chana's last statement had more than a ring of truth to it. Sometimes a woman is asked about her mother's labors, as a way to assess how her own birth experience might proceed. However, only half of our gene pool is from the maternal side, so it's a bit like we're only half-related to our mothers. But siblings share genes from both parents...so if a woman has sisters who've given birth, I'm always more interested in how those births went, rather than my client's mother's labor.

I had Carole's support as a midwife supervisor, and I had Bill's agreement to provide backup if needed, and I already had Sandi MacKenzie, an assistant/apprentice midwife whom I'd known for several years. According to her, she'd known I would become a midwife way before I had come to that conclusion, and she'd told her husband she was going to apprentice with me and eventually become a midwife herself.

So, to my surprise, I seemed to have everything in place, and now I had a client.

"You do realize," I said to Chana, just to be sure we were on the same page, "that I haven't graduated yet? I'm technically not a licensed midwife. A more experienced midwife will be present, too, plus my assistant, who is in training herself."

"Sounds great. Where do I sign up?"

Well. That was easy.

Chana and her boyfriend lived just half a mile from me, in a second floor apartment on Alcatraz Avenue – and yes, you can see Alcatraz Island in the middle of San Francisco Bay, straight ahead as you look west down the long street. As her due date was just a bit more than a month away, I made a home visit a few days later to begin to establish a relationship.

Upon meeting Lloyd, Chana's boyfriend and father of her baby, I realized that, as a couple, they made an unusual pair. Lloyd came downstairs to let me into the main door and escort me to their third floor apartment. At first glance, he looked very tired and a little dazed.

My next impression, as he sat across from Chana in their living room, was that perhaps he'd had too much to drink the night before and had a hangover. Drowsy expression, florid face, shabby clothing with a dirty shirt half-tucked. Mussed up hair, and he hadn't shaved that morning.

But as we began talking, I suspected that, in addition to alcohol, he might also be a drug user, actually maybe an addict. His bloodshot eyes had trouble focusing, and I noticed what looked like track marks on his exposed forearms. He slouched low in an armchair, scratched at a scab, and participated very little in the conversation.

I wondered what I'd gotten myself into.

Then Chana began to drive the dialogue, and I relaxed. She was clearly intelligent, well-educated, focused, and goal-directed. It was difficult to imagine how these two had ended up as a couple, but I found myself trusting Chana's judgment.

I made a second visit to the apartment a week later, and this time Lloyd wasn't present. Chana said he'd gone to do volunteer work at an animal shelter. I asked about his background, and she laughed.

"Everybody wonders what the heck we're doing together. Especially my father. He even offered to pay me a lot of money and set me up in a house in Palo Alto, where I grew up, if I'd agree to put Lloyd out of my life."

"Whoa," I said. "That's pretty...strong."

"Well, Lloyd's been in prison, and he uses heroin whenever he can get it. I don't think he's actually addicted again, like he was a bunch of years ago, but he's definitely not squeaky clean. Most of the time he's fine and when he uses it, he just goes to sleep. I mean, he's very sweet, and he's certainly not dangerous or anything."

"How did you two meet?"

"At the animal shelter. Him working there is part of his agreement with his parole officer – and we just hit it off. He's so kind, soft-spoken. He doesn't get up in my face about stuff like some other guys I've been with. I can be pretty strong and opinionated, and lots of guys can't deal with that. Lloyd is just easy to be with. And I know being with me makes it less difficult for him to deal with some of his issues."

I didn't pursue the topic. It wasn't my job to be their psychologist. Chana seemed to have things under control, so we proceeded with plans for her to give birth at home.

When Chana called me to say she was in labor, I could tell she wasn't active yet, but I went to the apartment anyway. She wore a T-shirt and panties, and was on her feet pacing from the bedroom to the living room and back again. Lloyd stayed at her side and held her gently as she rocked quietly with each contraction. Hours passed this way, and then it was morning. I went home to shower, change my clothes, and have breakfast with my family.

When I returned around 10:00 am, she was more active and beginning to make noise with her contractions. Sandi came around noon, and by the middle of the afternoon, Chana appeared to be in strong labor. I called Carole. She lived an hour away, and had a passel of her own children to corral, feed and shuttle here or there. She asked me how far dilated Chana was, so I examined her and wasn't surprised that she was nine centimeters.

"I'm on my way," said Carole, "as soon as I can get my husband home to take some of these kids off my hands."

I really hoped she'd make it in time, but I needn't have worried. Chana stayed at nine centimeters for more than four long and arduous hours. But she never once lost her perspective or her confidence, and, best of all, she never lost her sense of humor. Lloyd went to McDonald's at some point and returned with a bunch of hamburgers and fries. Chana had a few sips of a milkshake but wasn't interested in eating anything. Then, referencing the McDonald's catchy ad, she said, "I deserve a break today! This labor sucks. Really, don't you think so, guys? I deserve a break, dammit. I mean, *come on!*"

Carole finally arrived, and together we all decided that breaking Chana's bag of water might speed things along and give her the break she thought she so richly deserved. By then, she'd been stuck at nine centimeters for nearly five hours, and really, it was beginning to weigh heavily on all of us.

So I broke the waters, and wow! Almost immediately the baby dropped low into the birth canal and was born just half an hour later.

"Slow starters are often fast finishers," I said. "If you have another baby, I'm sure it'll be much easier."

They named the baby Leah.

* * *

I didn't hear from Chana again for ten years. When she called, I remembered every detail of her previous birth, as I think every midwife holds a special place in her heart for the memory of her first client's birth.

Chana and Lloyd had separated just before Leah's first birthday, but she said he made an effort to maintain contact and showed up now and then to spend an afternoon with Leah. Chana had received her Master's degree from Stanford. Two years earlier, she had married Robert, a Stanford professor of astrophysics and a self-described nerd. Out of his earshot, Chana whispered, "Brainiac, more like."

I had a "rule" that I didn't cross bridges to attend births. I didn't like to get too far from my base of support in Berkeley...but really, I just simply could not say No to Chana.

I drove toward San Jose and then across the bay on the Dumbarton Bridge and into Palo Alto, the town where Stanford University, also called The Farm, sprawls across its beautiful campus.

Chana and Robert's house was large and furnished sparely, very clean, modern, and super-organized. I made some comment comparing it to the dark and slightly dusty apartment where Chana's daughter had been born, and she laughed. "Things kind of turned out exactly like my dad hoped, in the end. Except he paid for my education rather than paying me to leave Lloyd. I split up with him when I finally realized he wasn't ever going to completely give up using drugs, and I needed to get both our daughter and myself out of that environment. Then I met Robert, and the rest is history."

"Is he behind the home birth plan?"

Robert, especially compared to Lloyd, was a pretty buttoned-up, serious-looking guy. He looked exactly like what he was: an academic, a professor at a prestigious university.

"Ha! It's taken me most of the pregnancy to get him on board. He's okay with it now, but only because I was like a dog with a bone on the subject. I'm pretty sure I'd have had all sorts of interventions with Leah's birth, you know, maybe even a Cesarean. No way in hell do I want to have this baby at a hospital, especially a university hospital where they have interns and residents practicing their new tricks."

"So no problems?"

"Nope. The only issue is he's not Jewish."

"Uh, what's the issue?" I knew Lloyd hadn't been Jewish either.

"Baby names. We've agreed on David, if it's a boy, but he wants to name a girl Rachel, and...well, I don't know how much you know about the Bible..."

"Not a lot, but I remember Rachel...and...her sister? Was Jacob in

19

there somewhere? Oh, I forget."

"Yeah, you're on the right track. Leah and Rachel were sisters, and there was all sorts of jealousy and envy between them. And trust me, it didn't end well. So, no way in hell am I'm going to have two daughters named Leah and Rachel."

"Well, Chana, you're on your own with that issue. Maybe it'll be a boy."

A few weeks later, Chana's labor started. Her waters broke shortly after contractions started, and I had a drive of about ninety minutes ahead of me, so I left immediately. I slid an audiocassette of Handel's Messiah into the tape player and let the majestic waves of music wash over me at top volume as I put the miles behind me.

Robert was fully present during the quick labor, but he was clearly dumbstruck at the drama of the event. I don't think anything in his previously well-ordered scientific life had prepared him for the magnitude of the situation. For how hard Chana would work. For how raw and visceral it all was. For how the birthing energy swelled in the room with each powerful contraction. Chana had been mostly quiet during Leah's birth, but this labor was much faster, much more relentless...and she roared like a she-bear.

"You definitely deserved a break last time, Chana, and you didn't get it," I said. "But today, you're getting that break. This time it's going fast for you."

"Really? It's not gonna last forever again?"

"Oh, no. Not a chance."

She didn't have time to answer before surging into another contraction.

Besides Margaret and me, it was Leah who did most of the hands-on help during labor; Robert held Chana's hand, but mostly he looked stunned, kept quiet, and just watched.

The infant surfed out on a wave of fluid that had been trapped in the uterus behind the baby's chunky body, and Robert yelped and jumped aside. I handed the baby to him and said, "Pass the baby up to Chana."

He did, juggling the slippery child for a moment, and as Chana took the infant, she said, "What is it?"

"I don't know," he said. "I didn't look. I don't care. I've never seen...I don't even...I can't...I...I don't have words."

Chana laughed, pulled a leg aside, and said, "Oh wow, it's another girl. Now we've got a battle on our hands. Sarah or Rachel. Do we have to fight some more about this, Robert?"

Robert stood up and raised his arms in total surrender. "Honest to God, I don't care. You can name her Sarah or Bathsheba or Hepzibah or Jezebel. After what I just saw you do, I figure it's totally your call. So, pick it, Chana. Just pick it."

They named her Sarah.

But they always called her Pickit.

But You're a Nurse, Right?

Delilah, another of my earliest home birth clients, called me a month before her due date.

I questioned how she'd found me, since I was still a couple of months shy of graduation. She, too, had found me through the ward clerk at Alta Bates, a woman who had suddenly become my biggest referral source.

"I have insurance," she said, "but I just took a tour of their labor rooms, and frankly, they're archaic. I can't imagine having this baby in what amounts to a big closet with just a bed and a steel toilet that pulls down from a compartment under the sink."

I'd seen those rooms, which have long since been demolished, and Delilah was correct: there was nothing inviting or warm-fuzzy about them.

I reminded her that I was still in midwifery school, technically not yet quite a midwife, and she said, "But you're an OB nurse, right?"

"Yeah."

"For like, forever, right?"

"Yeah, about fifteen-plus years."

"Well, then. I figure you've seen just about everything. You know what constitutes an emergency, right?"

"Yeah, of course."

"That's all I'm really interested in. Someone who knows it's still safe for me to stay at home. Provided everything stays on an even keel, nothing weird or dangerous is happening, I'll be fine at home, don't you think?"

Then she mentioned she was a nursing instructor at a local state university, and that really piqued my curiosity. I questioned her further, and she said, "I've worked in labor units, and it always seemed to me that, in the case of normal birth, the doctors were almost superfluous. The nurses really manage everything, and they're certainly well trained to recognize problems or any serious deviation from normal. Most of the time, it's like the doctor comes in at the end, catches the baby, and leaves. The OB nurses I've known could handle most things just fine on their own."

Well.

Really, I couldn't have stated it better myself.

Delilah and her husband, Joe, lived on a pedestrian walkway, in that there was no actual street – just a wide walking path between one side of the "street" and the other. Paths like these, usually with steep grades and several sets of crumbling stairs along the route, were designed to enable pedestrians to walk straight up or down a hill instead of having to go the long way round by following a curving street. Berkeley, Oakland, and San Francisco have many such paths, and they usually open onto scenic vistas toward San Francisco Bay. They also provide a traffic-free strip of space where children living in the houses along the path can safely play.

When Delilah's labor began, it was quickly clear she was one of those women blessed to have an efficient and no-nonsense labor with her first baby. I parked my little blue VW Bug with MITWIFE on the license plate out on the busy street at one end of the pedestrian path and schlepped all my gear to their house. Huffing and puffing a bit, I began to question the quaintness of these "short cuts" that provided no alternative to lugging grocery bags, baby strollers, suitcases, and midwife supplies by hand up and down steep paths and crooked stairways. When I arrived at the doorway of their Craftsman house, I felt a bit like a mule on an Alpine trail.

But the atmosphere inside the house was calm, though very busy. Sandi soon joined me, and we watched as Delilah navigated the second half of her labor by writhing and rolling around her large bed with slow and sinuous movements. She was an example of the axiom that, left to their own devices, many laboring women will shed one item of clothing for every couple of centimeters of dilation, rendering themselves entirely naked by the time they actually give birth.

I had called Carole Hagin earlier, and by the time she arrived, Delilah was nearly ready to push. She sprawled on the bed in repose between contractions, sometimes looking as though she were modeling for Goya's iconic painting, *The Naked Maja*. One arm stretched overhead, face turned to the side, back arched, one knee bent. Relaxed and peaceful.

Beautiful.

Carole, an artist in addition to all the other hats she wore, pulled a pen from her purse and began to sketch Delilah on the absorbent side of one of the slightly stained waterproof Chux pads lying on the bed.

The remainder of the birth was so straightforward that it could have been a textbook example of Normal.

Carole left shortly after we determined no stitching was needed. She wanted to get home to relieve her husband who, she said, was clueless in the kitchen. In spite of the fact that he and Carole were raising seven children together, she said, "He can do only two things for dinner: Kraft macaroni and cheese or order two large pizzas."

* * *

Three years later, Delilah called me again, pregnant with her second child. Again her labor was quick and efficient, perfectly normal. As I gathered my gear in preparation of leaving, I glanced up on the bedroom wall. And there, beautifully framed, was the Chux with the nude sketch Carole had drawn...with the smudged bloodstain clearly visible.

The Brown Leather Recliner

It's possible that Kitty elected to have her first baby at home in the hope that she wouldn't have to deal with any needles, but of course that hope was dashed on her first visit. When I handed her the lab slip for prenatal blood work, she turned white and began to wobble. Her husband steadied her, and the two of us guided her back to the exam table from which she'd just arisen.

"She hates needles probably more than anything else in the world," said Matt, her husband.

"Do you just want to get it over with, rather than having to worry about it?" I asked. "I can draw it here, right now, and then you won't have to stress about making an appointment later."

"And I won't have to take time off work to go with you," said Matt. "Yeah. Good idea. Let's just get it over with."

Kitty couldn't speak. Her eyes were wide and dark, like those of a lemur or some other little nocturnal jungle animal, and I'm sure her pulse was racing. Or perhaps it was slow as molasses and about to stop.

Mike looked at her for a response, but those eyes were locked on me in terror.

"Kitty! Kitty, just say 'Okay,' and it'll be over in a minute or two," said Matt.

Nothing.

"Maybe just nod your head a little?" he suggested, and we both saw the barest twitch of a nod.

Well.

It was a process, for sure. Matt leaned the weight of his whole body across hers, and I wondered if there was really a chance she would bolt upright and head for the hills with the needle dangling from her arm. Matt held her arm still with his left hand, kept her body in place with his own, put his face next to her ear and blathered on and on about who knows what. Meanwhile, with his free hand, he used his index finger to jab into the exposed skin on the arm I was about to stick with the needle.

As I applied the tourniquet and prepared to draw her blood as rapidly as possible, I asked Matt why he was poking her like that.

"It's worked before, like when we had to have blood drawn to get the marriage license. Maybe it distracts her or desensitizes her, I don't know, but it kind of worked that time, so I'm sticking with past success."

Still, when I stuck her with the needle, she shrieked and then went limp. I glanced up at her face. She didn't appear to have fainted; it was more like she was shell-shocked, just rigid and staring into space. The ABCs of CPR flashed through my mind, but I could see she was breathing, and when I touched her wrist with a fingertip, I felt a bounding pulse.

She just really, really didn't like needles.

I released the tourniquet, filled three tubes with blood, taking extra care not to let the needle wiggle in her vein as I switched from one tube to another, then put pressure on the puncture site with a cotton ball, pulled out the needle, and wrapped a piece of tape tightly around the spot.

Matt stood up. Kitty was free. Released. No one was touching her. But she just lay there as if she were in an eyes-wide-open coma.

I looked at Matt. "She'll come around," he reassured me. I checked her pulse again, which was fast but normal, then decided to let her lie on the exam table as long as she needed before daring to suggest she stand up.

So I moved on to another room to see my next client.

Half an hour later, I spied Matt supporting Kitty as she staggered out of the office. She was still pale, pale, pale.

Wow.

The thought that I'd need to draw her blood again in the third trimester was not something I wanted to think about at that moment.

Inevitably, it came time to repeat the blood draw when she was thirty-two weeks along, and Matt had invented a new twist to his system. Everything was the same as the previous time except that, in addition to poking at her arm with his fingertip, he sang some cowboy song loudly into her ear. It worked, and this time her post-needle trance was briefer, although they were the target of several surprised and curious stares as they walked out of the exam room. It was the song, I think, that had arrested everyone's attention – something about a man, his truck, his dog, and a faithless honky-tonk woman, as I recall.

An odd choice for the circumstances, but who was I to complain? The bloodletting was over.

It was Matt, not Kitty, who called me when labor began. Although I'd been attending home births for only a few months, I had already learned one of the axioms of the business: If the woman in labor calls, she's probably not very active yet, but if or when her partner calls, there's a good chance labor is running on all cylinders.

So I called Sandi, and we drove to the house together...and there sat Kitty in a brown leather rocking recliner, looking pretty much the way she'd looked right after I drew her blood, except this time her eyes were closed.

Wearing one of Matt's old T-shirts with a baseball theme, Kitty gripped the arms of the recliner tightly as she rocked back and forth, back and forth, back and forth. She made no noise at all, and except for seeing her belly round up into a hard little ball, I found it difficult to tell when a contraction began or ended.

Then Kitty threw up. Copiously. All down the front of her T-shirt. But she didn't stop rocking, and she didn't open her eyes. She just carried on as if nothing had happened. Matt ran to get another T-shirt while Sandi and I tried to clean her up – her hair, her chin, her lips, her neck – but she just kept rocking. She wasn't cooperating with our efforts to get the soiled shirt off her, and I could see that, without her help, we were going to make an even bigger mess trying to get the nasty-smelling thing over her head. So we just sopped up as much as we could, then wrestled a clean one over her head and pushed her arms through the sleeves...

And she rocked on.

Vomiting is fairly common toward the end of labor, so Sandi and I weren't surprised when Kitty's body began spontaneously pushing about half an hour after the whole throwing-up business. She was sitting well back in the depths of the recliner, sitting right on top of the spot where the baby would be coming out, but we needn't have worried. With a grunt and a heave, Kitty scooted her bottom forward to the front of the seat, and there was the baby's head for the three of us to admire.

That would be Matt and Sandi and me. Kitty still had her eyes closed.

And she was still rocking.

I caught the baby on the upswing, and she looked just like her mum looked after the blood draw: eyes wide open, pale, immobile, floppy…shell-shocked.

So, for the first time in my midwifery career, I performed CPR.

Well, really it was just PR, as her heartbeat was slow but still within normal limits. And in hindsight, the baby probably didn't need my help to initiate her breathing. The cord was intact, and the placenta was surely still doing its job. I maybe could have just waited, could have just given her time to get her act together on her own.

But it's hard to have a pale, limp, breathless, floppy newborn in your arms and not be inclined – indeed, feel compelled – *to do something*.

So I put my mouth over the baby's nose and mouth and puffed into her stunned looking little face. I could see Sandi attaching a re-breathing bag to my oxygen tank, but we didn't need it. As I was blowing in perhaps the fifth or sixth puff of air, the baby dramatically flew to life in my hands. Her arms and legs flexed and she battered both sides of my face furiously. Her body curled up like a little armadillo – and she screamed and screamed and screamed…right into my mouth.

One of the best sounds I'd ever heard.

Then we got down to the serious business of cleaning up the floor and the brown leather recliner. Kitty? Well, we put her in the shower, T-shirts and all. She stripped down, tossed the two wretched shirts out to us to throw away, and she washed her hair, her face, her ears, her chin, her neck…everything.

* * *

Two years later, Kitty and Matt had another baby. And yup, exactly the same scenario played out. The same silent, eyes-closed demeanor, the same brown leather recliner, the incessant rocking, the same vomiting issue, everything the same.

Except her second daughter needed no help whatsoever with being reminded that it was now her job to breathe on her own. She cried as soon as her shoulders were born.

* * *

Thirty-five years later, I was giving a book reading at a fundraiser in San Jose, California. About fifty women (and many nursing babies) attended, and at the end of the reading a tall, young blonde woman approached. She introduced herself, and I recognized her name from Facebook; it was Kitty's first daughter. And right behind her stood Kitty.

It was a sweet moment, and after we'd talked for five or ten minutes and had a few photos taken, I just had to ask:

"What about the brown recliner? Did you throw it away after your second birth?"

They looked at each other and laughed. "Oh, no," said Kitty. "It's practically taken on mythical significance. We definitely still have it."

"It's in my house now," said her daughter, "and sometimes I point to it and tell my boys that I was born right *there*. They say, 'In the recliner?' and look at me like I must be crazy."

Boose Gown Dooties

Oh, it was a long labor. We were sixty hours into it and still counting.

Ellen lived just a block from Alta Bates on a short street that had been truncated by the hospital's various expansion phases over the previous decades. Five families who owned vintage houses – two on one street, and three just around the corner on another street – had been affected by these changes to their quiet neighborhood, and they had bonded with each other. They did something that I've always thought was extraordinary with their properties: They formed a loose cooperative.

They tore down all hedges and fences that divided their backyards from one another, then planned and executed a complete restructuring of what now was to become common space. A single large barbecue and grill on its own patio would serve all the families. Narrow paths wove throughout the now quite large space for children riding their tricycles, and there was a sandbox and a climbing structure. A large vegetable garden and a separate flower garden were jointly cared for. One huge trestle table that could seat at least twenty sat in the center, but smaller tables seating two to six people were scattered here and there. While the flower and vegetable gardens were in almost full sun, old trees carefully preserved during the work phase provided plenty of shade over sitting areas. A few umbrellas covered some of the more exposed tables and lounge chairs. Several of the women did tai chi and yoga exercises on one of the small plots of grass.

It was utopia in action, a lovely urban communal "yard," and of course those involved in the planning and execution had become close to each other over the years.

And it felt like nearly all of them were involved in some way with Ellen's birth.

In addition to Pete, Ellen's husband, at least two women, not counting Sandi and me, were with Ellen at all times. As the hours wore on, they spelled each other, taking turns crooning to her, rocking and dancing with her, pacing down the hall, down the stairs, and then back up again. They held her arms as she swayed, they whispered encouragement into her ear, they brushed and stroked her hair. They showered with her. They kept all of us well fed and watered, and we each had the opportunity for an occasional nap.

Except Ellen, of course. She just labored on. And on and on and on.

As we rolled into evening and toward the second full night with no sleep, Ellen finally began to make progress a bit more quickly. The volume and intensity of some of the sounds she was making took on a more urgent quality. At one point, she turned and looked at my supplies laid out on a chest of drawers. Then she turned the other way and stared at the row of boxes lined up against the far wall – IV equipment, oxygen tank and re-breathing bag, extra Chux, gloves, gauze pads, and more – and she leveled a serious gaze on me.

"That's a lot of stuff," she commented.

"It seems like a lot to me, too, when I'm trying to get it all into someone's house in one trip," I said, "but it's really not that much, when you consider what they have in the hospitals for a normal birth."

"Yeah. Like drugs, right?"

"Sure."

"And are you sure, are you absolutely sure, that you don't have something for pain tucked away in even one of those boxes?"

Sandi and I smiled, and several of the women laughed aloud. Ellen gave them a look, they quieted down, and she turned back to me. "Nothing? Nothing at all?"

"Nothing. Sorry. I have no drugs for pain. This *has* been going on a long time, and the hospital's just around the corner. We can be there in less than five minutes if you feel like you've had enough."

"No, no. No, I was just asking, just curious. Just wondering… Kind of hoping maybe you'd been holding back when you told us you don't carry narcotics. No, as long as the baby is doing okay and I'm not in danger, I'll keep at it. I think of all those pilgrim women in the 1700s who did it, probably with a tenth of the support I have and certainly with none of the equipment you have. If they could do it, then surely I can do it."

So the hours rolled on.

Around eleven at night, Ellen moved into what appeared to be late labor, and she began a ritual of temperature management that drove the rest of us nuts. As each contraction began, she flung off her flannel nightgown and insisted that all the large windows be opened to the cold night air. But at the end of each contraction, we had to close all the windows again, and someone helped her slip the nightgown back on. Pete handled the window raising and lowering, while the women helped with the off-again, on-again nightgown routine.

It was winter, and it was raining. Soon, the room was frigid, and people went home, returning quickly with sweaters, blankets, and warm socks. But Sandi and I didn't have that luxury. So I called my husband and caught him just as he was about to head upstairs to bed.

"This woman wants four big windows wide open during each contraction, and we're all freezing. Can you please bring Sandi and me some cozy clothes?" I gave him the address, which was just a mile from our house.

"Sure. Some sweaters, sweatpants, stuff like that?"

"Yeah, perfect. And some warm socks."

"How about I bring your boose gown dooties? And maybe a couple of wool hats?"

That stopped me.

Boose gown dooties?

My husband has the endearing ability to utter unintentional and hilarious spoonerisms, the mixing-up of parts of words to create something that sounds like he's talking in code. This happens to everyone occasionally – but my husband does it more than just occasionally. And the oddest thing is that he goes right on talking instead of stopping to correct himself. It's as if he thinks if he just plows on ahead with the sentence, people won't notice.

Wrong.

"Boose…what?"

"What?" he asked. So now *he* was confused, too, and I realized he probably hadn't actually heard what he'd said.

"You said 'boose gown dooties.'"

"I did?"

"Yeah, and I'm working on it."

"Goose down booties. Your slippers."

"Of course," I said, and I laughed.

When I hung up, everyone was looking at me oddly. Sandi said, "Boose what? What's he bringing? Dooties? Some kind of a gown?"

"He meant to say goose down booties, but it came out wrong. Anyway, he's bringing a bunch of warm stuff for us that should hold us the rest of the night or however long this takes."

Ellen's labor never did truly speed up, but as the rainy skies cleared and a cold February sun began to shine, she finally felt like pushing. Three hours later, a nine-pound, dark-haired baby girl added her lusty cries to the tired shouts of joy and triumph that filled the room.

And finally Ellen settled on *warm* as her temperature of choice. We kept the windows closed, cranked up the heat, and warmed ourselves with mugs of thick hot chocolate as what seemed an endless supply of breakfast food began to appear.

And finally Sandi and I shed our down slippers.

But in our household – and between Sandi and me – they've always been, and always will be, boose gown dooties.

Across the Canyon

Gretchen was in labor with her first baby in a house perched on the rim of Claremont Canyon in Berkeley. Her bedroom window overlooked the cleft in the hillside, and we could see houses scattered among the pine and eucalyptus trees far on the other side of the canyon, maybe a quarter mile away as the crow flies.

The front door and entryway were at street level, but the rest of the house was built down the side of the steep hill, each of the four levels lower than the previous one.

Gretchen's bedroom was at the bottom of the house, and we had opened all the windows leading out to a wide balcony. It was a glorious afternoon in September, historically the month that boasts the Bay Area's best weather.

Labor had been progressing steadily, and Gretchen remained active and upright, pausing to lean against the wall or hang onto the shoulders of one of the several friends attending her birth. She sighed, she hummed, she moaned, and she sang little snatches of songs. It grew warm as the western sun angled into the room, dipping toward the horizon, and Gretchen stripped down to just a T-shirt and underpants.

In early labor, most women are chatty between contractions and breathe rhythmically during them. In mid-labor, women generally begin moaning or humming during the contractions. Then in transition, or late labor, everything gets turned upside down: a woman may fall asleep between contractions, then become noisy and behave very unpredictably during them.

Transition is usually part of a gradual trajectory, but for Gretchen, it came on like a race car shifting from second to fourth gear. Forget a pause for third gear. It slammed into her, full force, and we all knew the rest of her labor would probably be a wild ride.

She wiggled out of her underpants and yanked the T-shirt over her head as if both items were full of fire ants. Then she leaped onto the bed, stood upright, pressed her hands to the low ceiling – and she roared.

She roared a lot. She roared for quite a while.

She roared really, really loudly.

She didn't seem frightened or overwhelmed. She simply gave herself over to a power that was greater than anything she had ever experienced before. There was something decidedly primal and primitive about her sounds, and the rest of us just stood in awe of the raw energy that was manifest before us.

After about half an hour, I heard banging on the front door, three flights of stairs above us. It sounded as though the entire defensive line of the Oakland Raiders were trying to break into the house. I ran upstairs and opened the door.

Three cops, one with a gun drawn, stood there.

Then Gretchen roared again.

Both cops pushed past me and headed down the stairs.

"She's having a baby!" I yelled at their backs.

They stopped at the first landing, turned, and looked back up at me. "A baby? That's a woman in labor?"

"Yeah, a baby's coming. Jeez. Please, dude, could you put the gun away, at least? I'm the midwife, and she's in heavy labor. I know she's pretty noisy, but still. Just…uh, put your gun down. Please?"

"We got a lot of calls about somebody being attacked, maybe raped or murdered, somewhere up here in the hills." He holstered his gun before continuing. "All the calls came from the other side of the canyon, so it took us a while to locate you."

"She's fine. Really, she's fine."

"Um, well, we're sort of obligated to check. Just to make sure, you know? For our report?"

"Really?"

"Yeah, we need to just take a quick look?"

"Lord…" and off we tromped down all those stairs.

What they saw when they peeked around the corner and into the bedroom was a tall, very pregnant, very naked woman standing on the tousled bed. She was covered in sweat. Her long hair flowed over her shoulders, and her hands pressed against the ceiling like she was trying to hold the entire house up.

Then she roared again.

The cops didn't stay long.

The Birth Swamp

As I stood at the DMV counter waiting to renew my driver's license, I noticed a smudge high on my forearm. I wiped it, but when it left a sticky greenish-black smear, I knew what it was. Meconium. The sticky, tarry, dark stuff that constitutes the newborn's first poop.

I wrote "midwife" on the line asking for occupation, but figured if I wrote small enough, I could probably squeeze in "sanitation engineer," as well. I'd delivered Juliet's second baby earlier that morning, but I'd missed a spot near my elbow when I washed up afterwards.

Dealing with body waste is part of the job description when you earn your living catching babies. When women apologize for some unavoidable bodily function, I just smile and say, "Childbirth is life's great emptying event, and midwives always seem to be on the receiving end."

Just about every part of the body may give up its secretions during birth. Women sweat, cry, vomit, and drool. Their noses drip, and they spew spittle.

And that's the good news.

At the other end of the action, midwives are exposed to urine, blood, mucus, gas, and feces. Unless she's an artful dodger, the midwife frequently gets drenched with amniotic fluid when the bag of water breaks.

The Birth Swamp. That's what I sometimes call it, when things get especially messy.

Of course, some births are so bloodless and tidy that one needn't change the sheets afterwards. The vast majority fall between these extremes, but most definitely midwifery is not a profession for the squeamish.

However, when I drove up darkened Telegraph Avenue in Berkeley toward Bennett and Juliet's tiny Queen Anne cottage, I wasn't thinking of the janitorial services I might be performing. I expected only the joyful birth of a second baby. To avoid awakening her toddler upstairs, Juliet was laboring on the floor in her living room. Her bag of water broke just before dawn, and the fluid was as clear as Perrier water. However, only a trickle came out because her baby's head dropped and plugged the cervical opening. I knew there would probably be a big gush after the birth, so I gathered some towels, even made a little semi-circular dam to prevent overflow onto the rug.

Bennett was puttering around in the kitchen, and I smelled coffee and toast. Watery light trickled through tall bay windows. A wood-burning stove, Mission-style furniture, an antique rocker, and stained glass windows added an early twentieth century vibe to the tidy little room. Everything about this house and this birth spoke of cleanliness and peace.

By 6:00 am, Juliet felt like pushing. "Bennett, you'd better come," I said, knowing he wanted to catch the baby himself.

Bennett carried mugs into the living room, set them on the mantle, and stripped off his T-shirt. He removed his shoes and socks, then tied a bandana around his forehead to keep his long hair out of the way. Clad only in torn cut-offs and a faded headband, he looked like Tarzan – or a Sioux warrior.

Ready for whatever came next, he knelt between Juliet's bent knees. Turns out he was a lot better prepared than I was.

Juliet's damp hair straggled across her thin face as she strained into a push. Suddenly her bladder emptied in a little fountain, the urine whistling "ssssszzzzzz" under the pressure of her pushing. I grabbed a towel and held it to her crotch, but some hit Bennett and half a cup pooled between her legs.

He backed up for only a second, then moved into position again.

Juliet pushed her hair off her face and mumbled, "I feel sick."

As I reached for a wastebasket, she vomited a partly-digested burrito onto herself, Bennett, and into the urine puddle. I began wiping up with another towel, but my tidying efforts were interrupted by the appearance of the baby's head.

With her next push, meconium-stained amniotic fluid seeped around the edges of the head. This staining of the hind-waters, the trapped water still remaining in the uterus, alerted me that the baby had recently pooped. I soaked up the murky fluid with a third towel and pulled a suction catheter from my supplies.

Moments later, the head crowned. As Bennett leaned forward, concentrating on controlling the speed of the birth, a second arc of urine sprayed out, hitting his chest. He laughed and wiped himself off with a fourth towel.

The pile of soiled towels looked larger than my supply of clean ones. I dashed into the bathroom and grabbed all the towels from all the hooks – not exactly clean, but good enough.

Another contraction began. Suspecting the head would emerge this time, both Bennett and I leaned in close.

Juliet took a deep breath. But she didn't push. Instead, she launched herself into a sideways roll and landed on all fours, looking like a wild beast, a tawny tiger to match Bennett's Tarzan. Then she surprised us further by standing up and clawing at the wall as it she were scaling Yosemite's Half Dome.

Soldiering on, Bennett crawled forward, his knees sinking deep in the slimy puddle. Behind her now, he repositioned his hands on the baby's head.

Juliet sucked in another breath, then vomited again, this time splattering the cream-colored wall in front of her. Immediately the baby tumbled out, followed by at least a quart of the brown fluid I'd been expecting. It was heavily stained with meconium and very thick, the consistency of diluted peanut butter.

This was a colossal mess beyond all expectations. It was indescribable. It was epic.

My tidy dam of towels had long ago disappeared, and muck of all varieties overflowed the futon and the area rug, seeping relentlessly toward the edges of the room.

Juliet pressed her forehead to the wall and sighed, "Wow!"

"Yeah," I said. "Wow…"

Bennett, dripping with unspeakable filth, just grinned. "It's another girl!"

I blinked a few times. Then I waded into the swamp and dealt with mother and baby. When I'd suctioned the baby and checked that she and Juliet were both fine, I stared at the unbelievable scene, wishing I could call the fire department to come and just hose everything down.

Juliet burped, then hiccoughed.

"Oh, noooo," I moaned.

Bennett flinched.

Juliet vomited one last time. With that final heave, the placenta shot out and landed with a splash, followed by about a cup of blood. Amazed at the speed with which this quiet, calm, and pristine living room had been reduced to a scene of apparent carnage, I glanced at Bennett for his reaction.

Soaked from chest to toes, he still knelt in the primordial ooze. He held his hands out, staring at them as if they'd turned to gold. His eyes shone and his chest swelled with pride. As he spread his fingers, slime dripped from them.

"Wow," he breathed, echoing Juliet and me.

He wiped his fingers on his bare chest, leaving stripes of noxious gunk. As if applying war paint, he repeated the gesture on his forehead and cheeks. Grinning like a fool, he said, "This feels holy. Like something colossal to herald the dawn of the universe. I have the strongest urge to walk up to the French Café Bistro like this and order my morning latté."

All of Berkeley should be grateful he didn't act on that urge. Instead, he went outside and hosed himself off in the driveway. Then we spent two hours creating order once again in the living room. But the rug was trashed.

On my way home, I headed for the DMV, knowing it wouldn't yet be too crowded. I went from station to station with record speed, handed my completed application to the clerk, and had my picture taken.

When my new license came in the mail, I checked the photo. Not too bad. Then I looked closer. Yes, there was a tiny smear of something on my right cheek.

I knew exactly what it was.

Scream

Jane maintained her sweaty, claw-like grip on the sleeves of my black T-shirt. My neck still ached from the whiplashing she had just administered. She'd jerked my whole body forward and backward till I thought my gold crowns would shake loose. When she finally quit trashing me, I felt like a dizzy cartoon character. Only the stars, curlicues, and chirping birds drawn above my head were missing.

I needed the full two minutes of rest between her now ferocious contractions in order to recover my equilibrium.

Jane, who spent a full twenty-four hours of grueling labor progressing from one to three centimeters, had finally hopped onto the fast track. She was busy proving the truth, again, in the saying that slow starters can be fast finishers.

Fifteen minutes earlier, her face had transformed with a startled stare of newfound knowledge. A switch flipped, and she saw The Way. Her Way. She latched onto my shirt and began screaming with her damp cheek pressed to mine. Throughout the whole contraction, she yanked me every which way from Sunday as she screamed into my ear.

The first stanza was a brief preamble: "Uhh-*ah!*" with a lilting upturn of volume on the second syllable.

She held the second stanza about twice as long as the first. Louder, too.

Finally came a long, sucking intake of air, a pause at the top in which time stopped. Then came the real deal. A scream to put all other screams to shame.

I didn't know a human could make such a sound. I didn't know a woman in labor could scream that long without taking a breath. She held that solitary, hair-raising, high-octave pitch without a single waver in her voice for the entire duration of the strongest part of each contraction.

It set my eardrum vibrating in the aural equivalent of an epileptic fit.

When it finally ended, I said, "Jane, we have to have a little chat."

I knew I'd spoken, but I couldn't hear myself or anyone else. I shook my head like a terrier with a foxtail in its ear, and the residual humming died down at last.

Jane listened to my speech of how low, back-of-the-throat noises work better than high-pitched screams, how the deeper tones are more relaxing than the shrieks, how matching moans and sighs to slow, sinuous, rocking movements help put mind and body on the same wave length.

A glimmer of hope and trust replaced the glazed look of terror in her eyes. I thought I'd gotten to her, and I thought perhaps, just perhaps, my hearing could be saved.

No such luck.

She tried, she really did, but hysteria greeted each attempt to keep her voice low, and it quickly became obvious that, for Jane, only screaming at top volume while thrashing somebody about like a wet mop in a tornado, was going to work.

We sighed but we figured if we rotated players in this drama, no one person would be overly assaulted. So Sandi took my place for a couple of the contractions, but Jane said, "Too little, too thin."

Jane's husband, Mike, took Sandi's place, but Jane pushed him away. "Too big. Oh, way too big."

Her sister and her best friend each took a turn, but Jane whined, "Wrong shirt" to her sister and "Too much hair" to her best friend.

"I want Peggy. *Please*, I just want *her!*"

Ouch.

I stuffed my ear with wads of Kleenex. Kneeling in front of Jane, I wished for something more effective than Kleenex, but noise-cancelling headphones hadn't been invented yet. The next hour seemed like the longest hour of my life, but thank goodness that's all it took for Jane to zoom to complete dilation.

Then, just as suddenly as it had started, her screaming stopped. She settled into a sweaty squat and pushed in absolute silence, needing only thirty minutes to give birth to a nine-pound baby boy.

Fifteen minutes later, the young couple who lived in the upstairs apartment knocked on the door. Bearing a tray with coffee, orange juice, and fresh cranberry scones, they crept into the bedroom, open-mouthed in awe.

"We *heard*," they said.

"I'll bet you did," said Mike.

At least that's what someone told me later. For two days, I couldn't hear a thing.

Black Bean Soup

Donna was planning a home birth, but it was destined to be a marathon, not a sprint. She labored on and on and on.

Sandi and I got hungry and began foraging in the refrigerator and cupboards.

The almost-empty fridge held milk and lettuce, a bottle of ketchup, a jar of mustard, some orange marmalade, and pickles. We checked the cupboards and found sugar, salt, an onion, and a few basic spices.

Feeling a little desperate, we peered into the freezer. One pound of Peet's coffee beans, half a carton of mocha chip ice cream, and two quarts of frozen black bean soup stared back at us.

That's pretty much all there was to eat in the house. Really.

No cereal. No bread, peanut butter, or jam. No eggs or cheese. No vegetables.

Worst of all, no chocolate.

Sandi looked me and whispered, "What do you suppose they eat?"

I shrugged. She began thawing the black bean soup while I fetched two spoons from a drawer, and we quickly ate most of the ice cream.

Several more hours passed. Donna's labor slowed way down, stalled, then totally stopped. We walked her, did nipple stimulation, stretched her cervix...every trick we could think of to get labor to kick in again.

Finally, she started contracting, and Sandi and I were just on the verge of phoning in an order for a ginormous pizza loaded with everything – or maybe a triple order of sushi – when Donna's bag of water broke. You could hardly call it "water." It was thick with meconium. I've never understood why unborn babies don't empty their bowels regularly before birth. I mean, why save it all up? But save it up they do...unless something happens to distress them, which leads to a relaxation of the rectal sphincter.

If the amniotic fluid is only lightly or even moderately stained, most midwives don't become too concerned, provided the baby's heartbeat behaves itself. We monitor the baby more closely and prepare for some serious suctioning when the baby is delivered, but that's about it.

But when meconium is as thick and dark as Donna's was, it's called "pea soup meconium" and I knew we should be in the hospital. This was not a baby I wanted to deliver at home. Donna would receive continuous fetal monitoring and, after the birth, the baby would receive more targeted suctioning than we were equipped to do at home. If something serious was causing distress or the baby needed the resuscitation team, then the hospital was clearly the place we needed to be.

And indeed, something was distressing Donna's baby. Its heartbeat slowed during the contractions and took its own sweet time climbing back up to normal after her contractions ended. The rate wandered between one hundred, too low, to one hundred sixty, the upper limit of "normal."

* * *

Bill Stallone and his wife, Laura, had been my first backup doctors. When they closed their Bay Area practice and relocated to Southern California, Dr. James Jackson offered to provide backup for both Carole and me. We also paid him a pittance, for he would accept no more, to rent two exam rooms in his office in which to hold our clinical office hours two days a week.

Late in his life, as I sat at Dr. Jackson's bedside after he had entered hospice care, we had several long discussions about his early life.

"Why did you offer to back me so readily?" I asked, as we were remembering those days thirty years earlier.

"I was born at home," he said, "so I've always had a soft spot for midwives and doctors who are willing to put themselves on the line and deliver babies at home. My mother lived in rural Georgia, and there was only one doctor who was willing to care for black women. He lived at the parsonage, and my mother told me she had a very fast labor with me. She said, 'That doctor ran across the fields and jumped a fence to make it in time for your birth.'"

"What a great story," I said, and I reached out and squeezed his thin brown hand. He was a gentleman, and I don't recall that he ever treated anyone – patient or nurse or doctor – with anything other than kindness, respect, and compassion.

* * *

So I made a phone call to Dr. Jackson, alerted him to the fact that we were heading into the hospital and told him the important details of the situation: meconium in the fluid, the baby's iffy heartbeat, and the desultory labor pattern.

"See you soon," he said.

Donna's husband, Sandi, and I began packing up and ferrying stuff outside to our various cars. While we were occupied, and unbeknownst to us, Donna wandered into the kitchen, where, when I went looking for her, I found her shoveling a huge chunk of still partly-frozen thick bean soup directly into her mouth.

"Oh, no, no, no," I said, running to stop her. I took away the spoon and plastic container and asked, "How much did you eat, Donna?"

"What, what?" she asked, reaching for the container with both hands.

"It's not likely, but in case there's an emergency and they need to operate quickly, by putting you to sleep, it's way better if you're stomach's empty," I explained, hurrying her along. "How much of it did you eat?"

"Um, the rest of the ice cream and probably a cup of the soup. Maybe more."

I sighed.

It was my fault for not warning her about not eating, especially since I'd begun to suspect she might end up with a Cesarean. But it just hadn't occurred to me that she would choose exactly this moment to chow down on black bean soup and ice cream.

On the other hand, there really wasn't much else in the house to eat. Lettuce, maybe? With mustard?

"They're not going to be very happy about this when we get to the hospital, but they'll deal with it. They'll have to. Let's go."

At the hospital, a nurse attached a fetal monitor to Donna. The paper strip recording the heart rate of the baby and the strength of the uterine contractions showed that Donna's contractions were weak in quality and five minutes apart. The baby looked sort of okay, but Donna was dilated only halfway, and we all knew we had a long road ahead of us with a baby whose reserves appeared to be marginal.

Dr. Jackson stopped in to introduce himself and to evaluate Donna's condition. After a brief discussion, we started Pitocin. Quickly, the contractions picked up in intensity and frequency, but the baby's heart rate took a nosedive. And the ominously thick meconium continued to spill out.

It became clear to everyone that we were headed for a Cesarean.

While Dr. Jackson was scrubbing for surgery, the anesthesiologist came into the labor room for a pre-op interview. He introduced himself, poked around on Donna's back to check for possible placement of a spinal needle, then asked the routine question I'd been dreading.

"When did you last eat?"

Oh, boy, I thought. Here it comes.

Donna glanced at the clock, then said, "About three hours ago."

"Hmm. And what did you eat?"

"Mocha chip ice cream."

"And black bean soup," chimed in her husband. "But the soup was still mostly frozen," as if that somehow made it okay.

The anesthesiologist turned and stared at me.

"I know, I know. She got into the kitchen when I wasn't looking."

"Black bean soup," he repeated.

"And the ice cream," prompted Donna.

"Right." The anesthesiologist was still staring at me. "Bean soup. Great."

"At least we're not lying about it," I said. It was kind of a lame rebuttal, but it was all I could come up with.

"Well, yes. There is that. At least I'll know what to be prepared for."

Fortunately there was no problem. Donna was able to have a spinal, not a general. And she didn't vomit. But if she had, the anesthesiologist would have been prepared to suction her so she didn't aspirate chunky black beans into her trachea, which could have been disastrous.

As Donna and her baby were being wheeled to the Recovery Room, the anesthesiologist looked at me again and shook his head. "Bean soup. Lord."

Moral to the story to midwives of the future: Black bean soup is definitely not the best choice of food for a woman in labor, but if the mom eats something weird, don't try to lie your way out of it if you end up at the hospital. It's not often a problem, but when it is, it can be very serious.

Aztec

Jessica came to me wanting a home birth for her second child. At our first visit, she hugged me, greeting me like an old friend. She reminded me that I'd been her nurse when she'd had her first baby in the Alta Bates Birth Center.

I really couldn't quite place her. After all, it had been four years, and I'd seen hundreds of births in the intervening years.

But I didn't want to hurt her feelings. So I didn't admit I'd actually forgotten the details of her birth.

I did a prenatal home visit when she was in her last month of pregnancy, and she brought out an album of photos from the birth. We looked at the pictures together, and sure enough, I had definitely been present.

But still, nothing really rang a bell.

So she progressed through the pregnancy...and I continued allowing her to think I had vivid memories of the birth of her four-year-old child.

She labored very quickly second time around, maybe five hours total. When I arrived, she was lying in bed. Unlike most women, she seemed to prefer staying there, rather than walking around the house, leaning against the walls, hanging from other people's shoulders. She sat cross-legged in bed, propped up with eight or ten pillows surrounding her, and she hummed quietly, lightly drew circles on her belly with her fingertips, and smiled through all but the last few minutes of her labor.

When Jessica began pushing, the baby came quickly and easily, at least from my perspective. About fifteen minutes after the birth, she handed the baby over to her husband, stood up naked, and began walking to the bathroom for a shower.

"Aha!" I said as I watched her walking away from me.

She turned and looked at me oddly. "What?" she asked.

"I'd forgotten about that calendar," I explained, and she shrugged and went on into the bathroom.

But as soon as I saw her butt, the whole experience of four years earlier rushed back to me in exquisite detail.

Yes, a calendar on her butt triggered an entire intact memory of that previous birth. It was…distinctive: an incredibly detailed and very large tattoo of the famous Aztec calendar covered her entire right bum cheek.

Her mother had been present for that birth in the hospital. Back then, when Jessica got up to go to the bathroom afterwards, she wrapped her gown tightly around her body before walking away. But when she turned into the bathroom, with me following behind, the gown fell open, and I saw the tattoo for the first time.

"Whoa. Wow, let me see that!" I said, leaning in for a closer look at the astonishing and delicate job.

"Sssh," she hissed, whispering to me.

"What?" I said.

She peeked around the corner to make sure she was out of her mother's line of sight. "My mom doesn't know I got this tattoo done, and now is not the time to show her, I don't think."

I laughed, helped her with her shower, then slipped one gown on covering the front of her body and a second gown worn backwards that covered her from behind. Protected from her mother's discovery, Jessica's tattoo was thoroughly under wraps when she reentered the birth center and began nursing her daughter.

So four years had passed. I assumed this amazing tattoo was no longer a secret. But as Jessica returned to the bedroom after showering, she turned to me and said, "You know, my mom still doesn't know I have this thing, and I'd like to keep it that way. She's due to arrive within half an hour. So everybody? Just remember. *Bum's the word!*"

Wrong Restaurant

"She said she farts every time her baby punches her low in her belly. It's turning into a serious social problem, and she asked me what to do about it."

Carole Hagin related this tidbit from her morning in prenatal clinic to Sandi and me as we stood in the lobby of an upscale restaurant, waiting for Ming, Carole's new partner to join us. Sandi and I yelped with laughter, and the carefully-coiffed hostess raised her eyebrows at us.

Carole and I were figuring out the details of covering each other for vacations and for those "full moon" occasions when more women were in labor than either of us could manage on our own. Otherwise, we were on call at all times for our own clients. I had Sandi working with me, and Carole was joining up with Ming, a Chinese midwife with years of practice in her native country. We all expected to gain from her experience.

"Here she is," said Carole, and Sandi and I turned and watched a late-model Audi park next to Carole's rusty sedan with a bungee cord holding the trunk closed. She always said her husband brought stray cars home the way other people took in stray cats, and her car was living proof.

Ming stepped out of her shiny car, and I looked at her curiously. I knew only that she was a Chinese midwife, highly skilled in everything except her mastery of English. She was tall, taller than any Chinese woman I'd ever met. She wore no makeup, and her hair looked as if it had been cut in the same shop where the Chinese students on San Francisco's cable cars had theirs cut: razor straight bangs and the sides bobbed just below her ears.

We were still laughing about Carole's farting client when Ming came inside. After we'd done the introductions, Ming asked, "What funny?"

"Carole has this woman who farts every time her baby kicks," I said quietly.

Ming covered her mouth with the tips of her fingers and laughed shyly. "Oh ho ho, and what you say?" she asked, looking at Carole.

"Well, she caught me off guard, and all I could think to offer was the suggestion that she carry room deodorizing spray at all times, perhaps a nice floral scent."

The hostess cleared her throat, and we swallowed our laughter.

Conversation between midwives is often bawdy, and I was delighted to see that, in spite of her somewhat formal manner, Ming laughed along with the rest of us. I thought this boded well for our relationship and the future of our loosely connected clinical practices. And it was certainly a good opening for our first meeting all together.

With 20/20 hindsight, we later agreed that particular restaurant wasn't the best choice for this meeting. We should have picked perhaps a noisy Berkeley bistro on Telegraph Avenue, one like Bateau Ivre, with outdoor seating and lots of traffic noise to block some of our conversation. But Carole had chosen a quiet restaurant in Lafayette, a conservative suburban community. The restaurant with a French name was convenient for all of us, but the ambience was proving to be a possible problem.

Tapping the reservation list with manicured fingertips, the hostess looked down her nose at us, a giggling motley crew compared to the other guests. Large bouquets of lilies and delphiniums graced the entryway, and a Vivaldi violin concerto drifted from invisible speakers. As our shoes sank noiselessly into pale jade carpeting, we tried hard to match our behavior to our surroundings.

Soft silks, pastels, pearls, thin belts, and cashmere cardigans clothed the thin and elegant bodies of women at nearby tables. Dressed in Guatemalan print shirts, denim, and 100% cotton Earth First T-shirts, we probably looked like aliens to the other guests, and we were certainly aware of their glances our way. Ming, dressed in tailored navy and white, represented our best chance for blending in, but she looked more like a waitress than a guest.

I took a deep breath and picked up the small menu, hand-written in lilac ink on thick vellum. I caught Sandi's eye, but it was too soon to trust an exchange of glances. We quickly looked away, and I bit my cheek to stop another round of giggles.

As two women at an adjacent table said something about "a silk wrap" as they compared fingernails...well, I swear the devil made me do it. I said, "Funny, I don't hear anyone else talking about room deodorizers in here."

Collectively, we lost it. As we laughed, heads turned our way. In another era, eyepieces would have been raised to allow them to get a better look at us.

Giving us a sliver of a smile, no more, the server came to take our orders.

After she'd retreated, Carole asked, "Do they throw people out of places like this for having too much fun?"

"I think we're pushing some buttons," said Sandi.

"What means 'push buttons'?" asked Ming, and we tried to explain.

"Ah, so much to learn. So much funny things you say. I need listen and learn."

When our food arrived, Carole looked at her small individual prosciutto pizza and chuckled. "I've been meaning to tell you guys about this. A couple of weeks ago, I delivered a baby, and the placenta was really..."

"Carole, shhh," cautioned Sandi as at least ten pairs of eyes pivoted toward us at the word 'placenta'.

"Right. Sorry, sorry." Carole leaned toward the middle of the table and we bent closer to hear her. "Anyway, this woman had what looked like two complete p-l-a-c-e-n-t-a-s, separated by about three inches of membrane with three blood vessels running across the gap. I wanted to share it with the midwifery students, so I took it home, spread it on a cookie sheet, covered it with foil and froze it."

"Sheet? For bed?" asked Ming, looking confused.

The idea of a placenta spread out like a sheet on a bed made us snort into our lunches as Ming whispered, "What is cookie sheet?"

Carole explained what a cookie sheet is, then continued. "One of my sons had friends over, and they got hungry. He lifted the edge of the foil, thought it was a pizza, and popped it into the oven at 400 degrees."

"Oh no no no no no," whispered Ming, covering her mouth with both hands.

"Oh yes yes yes yes yes," said Carole. "The boys were expecting a cheesy garlicky aroma, and instead the house began to reek of something like liver and kidneys. One of the guys said, 'It smells like cat piss in here. What the hell is that?'"

"Shhh," I whispered.

Carole lifted her pizza and took a bite, then tilted her head back in pleasure and moaned, "Ummm, placenta with prosciutto. My favorite."

Our laughter sputtered again, but then Ming said, "Sorry, what means pro-shitty?"

"Prosciutto!" hollered Carole, and we were lost.

The restaurant was very quiet – except for us. The hostess stared at us. A man in a three-piece suit emerged from an office and peered at us over the top of his glasses. With great difficulty and a huge dose of self-control, we swallowed our bubbling laughter and got through the rest of the meal by strictly censoring the subject matter.

After dividing the bill and leaving a huge tip as penance, we waited for our receipt. Carole asked me, "Are you still teaching birthing classes?"

"No, it got too stressful. I was always fearful I'd have to cancel a class on short notice to attend a birth."

"I noticed something when I used to teach," Carole said. "When I taught the class on pushing, someone always farted. Did you ever notice that?"

"Well, occasionally…," I answered, aware of the server heading our way with the credit cards and receipts.

"I swear it happened every time. But here's the thing. It was the guys who were doing almost all of the...

"....farting," she finished, just as the server came alongside us.

Sandi collapsed forward, resting her head on the table. I rocked from side to side, hugging my ribs. Carole bellowed with laughter, and her nose turned bright red.

Ming said, "But what is…," then turned red and just stared at the ceiling.

"Oh dear lord, we've got to get out of here," I mumbled. We leaped to our feet and hurried to the lobby. Wringing her hands, the hostess behind the enormous floral bouquet said, "Ladies, ladies…"

"We're leaving, we're leaving," said Carole.

"Right now," I said.

"Sorry, sorry," mumbled Sandi.

"But what is…?" stammered Ming, bringing up the rear, but Sandi grabbed her arm and pulled her toward the door.

Ming stopped and said, "Wait, please wait," so we all quieted down and turned to her in silence. We had the attention of the entire restaurant, and the silence was deafening.

Into the silence, Ming said clearly, far too clearly, "But, wait. Please to tell me. What means 'farting'?"

We never went back.

Shall We Call My Parents?

Sharon's first baby had taken a long time to come into the world, but most people know that subsequent labors can be very different. A long first labor is no indication, really, of what pattern the second baby's birth might follow.

Midwives have a saying: First labors are long. Second labors are short. Third labors are unpredictable.

Of course, it's really a toss-up each time. But still.

When Sharon's husband called me at one in the morning to say labor had been underway for a couple of hours, I drove to their house in the Berkeley hills right away. Her contractions were fairly close, about three minutes apart, but her cervix was dilated only about the width of a nickel. I checked all the vital signs and then told them, rather than returning home and waiting for them to call me later, I'd bed down with their dog in the living room for a while.

"Wake me in a couple of hours, okay? But of course wake me up if you have any questions, if you need something, or if your labor pattern changes... Anything at all, right?"

They agreed, and I grabbed a couple of pillows and a blanket and curled up on a couch in the corner of the living room. Their large black Labrador flopped next to me, pressed against my back.

I had been asleep for no more than an hour when I was suddenly and completely alert. Something had awakened me abruptly, but as I sat staring into the darkness, all was silent.

I waited.

Then I heard it again: "AAAA-OWWW-OOOOO..."

I threw off the blanket, stumbled over the dog, and raced into the back bedroom. The dog's toenails click-clacked on the bare wooden hallway floor as he ran right behind me.

Sharon and her husband were sitting cross-legged on the bed. They stared at me in silence, looking mildly curious at my sudden appearance.

I said, "What was that noise?"

Stupid question, I know, for I knew full well what that noise signified, but I was groggy and besides, they were reading the Sunday New York Times. They sat side by side, propped up in bed, newspapers spread out all around them, and they were sipping tea.

They both looked entirely composed.

They frowned. "What noise?" they said in unison.

"Something like 'AAAA-OWWW-OOOOO'..." I mimicked, feeling as though I was trying to impersonate a hound dog that had just treed a possum.

"Oh, yeah, Sharon sounded something like that with the last contraction, I guess."

I checked her, and she was almost fully dilated.

When I told her, Sharon's jaw dropped open. "Really? But wait. Should we call my parents? Will they have time to get here?"

"Probably, if they hurry. How far away do they live?"

"New York."

My mind raced...was there a town somewhere in California, preferably close to Berkeley, called New York? I'd never heard of it, but hey, I'm human. I don't know everything.

"New York? New York City? As in, Manhattan? Central Park? New York, where the Empire State Building is? The New York that's three thousand miles away?"

"Yes. They came when labor started with my first baby and arrived with plenty of time to spare. We just wanted to be sure this was really labor before we called them this time. They live pretty close to the airport and have an open ticket. Will they make it?"

"No."

Gains and Losses

I gained so much richness in my life by becoming a midwife, and those gains became apparent very quickly.

I gained autonomy. I was no longer obligated to follow doctors' orders I didn't agree with. I became the one writing the orders. When a woman began pushing, I could allow her to take as long as she needed, provided both she and baby remained in good condition. No one was looking over my shoulder with a figurative stopwatch, telling me that just because two hours had passed and still the baby hadn't been born, then she should have a Cesarean.

I gained the ability, as much as possible, to choreograph a woman's ideal birth. If she wanted to have thirty-five neighbors present, if she wanted her husband or her sister or her teenage daughter to catch the baby, if she wanted a water birth...these things were possible, even in the hospital.

At home births, there were even more creative choices for a laboring woman. She could eat rhubarb pie during labor, she could burn candles or incense, she could have her dog – or dogs – beside her the entire time. She could bake cookies during active labor, walk from tree to tree in her backyard, or ask all twenty members of her long-standing women's group to come at the last minute. She could, as one of my clients actually did, invite the mailman to come inside and watch.

I could help restore a woman's faith in herself and her body by supporting her through a vaginal birth after a previous Cesarean. This was especially gratifying and fulfilling to those women who suspected the Cesarean had been done too hastily or unnecessarily, cheating her of the birth experience she'd hoped for. I could watch healing take place right before my eyes.

When it was necessary to move a woman from home to hospital, I could make the unwanted or unexpected transition as smooth as possible, and I could remove barriers to continuity of care. The nurses were supportive of me, and this support extended to my clients. My backup doctors didn't have ego problems with the fact that some women preferred a midwife to a doctor. They always responded when I needed them and never made me feel as though they questioned my judgment.

One gift I received over and over came from some of my patients themselves. The determination of women giving birth for the first time who chose to do so at home never ceased to humble and awe me. They didn't know what contractions would feel like, but they believed they would manage them. They knew pain medication wasn't an option, but they believed they wouldn't ask for it. They couldn't imagine the unbelievable sensation of the vaginal opening stretching wide, wide… and then just a little bit wider to allow the passage of a baby's head.

But they trusted. They trusted their bodies and themselves to achieve this seemingly impossible feat. And they trusted me to help them through the rough spots.

Blind faith in knowing they were joining the ranks of women from past millennia who had all somehow "done it" led them to trust themselves and the birth process to a degree that I had not been capable of myself when I was pregnant with my own first child.

Admittedly, these first-timers were usually blown away by how hard birth is, how much it hurts, how long it can sometimes last…yet they did it. And I had the honor of seeing their faces turn toward me as they held their newborns in their arms, faces transformed by a new awareness, a sense of accomplishment, a feeling of disbelief…

And I watched as they stepped across an invisible but definable threshold. I watched each one change from Girl to Woman.

And then to Mother.

I deeply admired them – and still do. It was profound, and it brought tears to my eyes. Every single time.

But there were also losses.

The most practical of the losses included a steady and predictable paycheck, paid vacation, health benefits, and sick time. I gave up a job with regular hours on the day shift, the certainty that I could sleep all night, and the ability to promise my children I would be home on Christmas morning.

There was another loss. A poignant one. One I didn't anticipate. I failed to appreciate how much I would miss handing over one part of my role as nurse to another person when I switched from being nurse to midwife: the exquisite pleasure of feeling a baby leave the mother's body.

As a midwife, I was busy at the action end of things, and I missed this sweet sensation...

A woman is straining, working as hard as she can
to push her baby into the world.
I place my palm softly on her belly, but I don't feel
much of a difference when the head is born.
So I wait, I wait sometimes for three or four minutes
until the next contraction begins.
As the first shoulder appears,
the alignment of the baby's body shifts,
and I feel a little bum rise upward to fill my cupped palm.
With the delivery of the second shoulder,
the baby's bum dips again toward the mother's spine.
And then, oh, quick! I must be quick, or I'll miss it.
I must look and feel at the same time...
As the baby's body emerges into the world,
changing like malleable clay on a potter's wheel
from an amorphous bump in a belly
into a baby alive in the world,
there is a moment when my hand on that belly
actually feels the body leave the uterus.
The last sensation is that of the legs straightening out
for the first time,
and I feel a brief flutter kick as of a tiny swimmer
pushing off from the side of the baby pool.
And then it's gone.
There is nothing beneath my hand.
But from just a foot or two away,
there is the sound of a newborn's cry.

I was raised a High Church Episcopalian, and while I am no longer conventionally religious, more than once as I felt this transformative process occur beneath my hand, I recalled a verse from the old King James Bible:

*"And the Word was made Flesh and dwelt among us,
full of grace and truth."*

Yes, we know, intellectually, that there's a whole living baby dwelling inside the womb, but it's really hard to believe. It feels as though it must be a conjurer's trick, arranged somehow with smoke and mirrors.

Interestingly, the person in the room who seems most surprised at the moment of birth is the woman who has carried this child within her body for the past nine months. The woman who has been working hard for who knows how many hours to bring this baby Earthside.

Too many times to count, I've heard women exclaim, "Oh! A baby!"

Once, a new dad stared at his wife in astonishment as she uttered this comment, and he said, "Well, yeah. What did you expect? A standard poodle?"

But yes. Incredible as it seems at the end, it's a baby. It really is.

And that is always a plus.

Mailman

A woman's freedom to craft the birth of her dreams is greatly increased when she chooses a midwife to attend her birth. And that freedom soars even higher when she decides to give birth in her own home. Limited only by the bounds of safety, really, anything goes.

But not everyone invites the mailman to come in for the occasion.

Belinda lived in a modest two-bedroom house in Berkeley's flatlands, and by the time her second baby was about to be born, the house was jammed with friends, neighbors, and family members. The little home sat in a cluster of six identical houses arranged symmetrically on a single piece of property along both sides of a wide walkway that ran perpendicular to the street...a bit like summer cottages might be positioned close together with a common area between them where children and dogs could safely play. Almost of necessity, the families in those six houses had grown close over the years. They babysat for each other's children, shared working in the gardens, had regular potlucks and barbecues...and now they had all been told they were welcome to come along for Belinda's Birth Ride.

And they all came. At least, it seemed that way to me. There were a lot of them. A whole lot.

They brought children, casseroles, pies, cameras, and wine. Sausages and ribs sizzled on a large grill across the walkway. They brought gifts for the newborn and gifts for Danny, who would soon be a big brother. They brought smiles, laughter, jokes, and quiet conversation.

There were so many bodies that the bedroom overflowed, and people in the hallway couldn't see. Children wiggled between the legs of adults and crowded around the bed. One little fellow climbed onto the bed and began jumping, but adult arms caught him mid-air and lifted him out of the way.

As she looked around at the crowd, Belinda realized we'd definitely outgrown the bedroom. She looked at me and said, "How much time do I still have?"

"Can't say exactly, of course, but probably less than half an hour."

"So, we've got time to move, right?"

I didn't catch her drift.

"Move?" I asked, thinking she meant she wanted to go to the hospital. But that didn't make sense: she was doing great, not complaining, barely making any noise above a low humming sound at the peak of some of the stronger contractions. "Move where? Do you mean the hospital?"

"No, no. God, no, not the hospital. No. I'm thinking we should move this show into the living room so everyone has a little room to breathe. Do we have time?"

"Sure," I said, but it was quite a process. There were people everywhere, and getting all my gear gathered up while maintaining some semblance of sterility for a few of the important bits and pieces, plus the oxygen tank, the IV box, the emergency supplies...it wasn't going to be easy.

Belinda's husband solved the problem. "Okay, dudes! Hey! Everybody leave and go wait in the courtyard. Then we can move into the living room, get ourselves organized, and y'all can come back inside."

In an organized little parade, everyone filed out. They stood outside in the sunshine, sipping wine, nibbling cheese, and holding babies on their hips while inside, I rearranged the principal players in the far more spacious living room.

And the room filled up again.

Once resettled, Belinda started to act like the baby was ready to come. A thick rope of bloody mucus clung to her thigh. The bag of water broke with a gush, and she was ready.

Then someone knocked on the open door, and we all turned to see who it could be. Surely everyone who planned on being there was already present.

It was the mailman.

He saw only a crowd of people and probably assumed there was a party going on. Well, there *was* a party going on, of course, but no doubt not the kind he was thinking of.

"Got a package that needs to be signed for," he said.

"Uh, can you come back later?" said the woman with a baby on her hip. "We're having a baby right now, and..."

"A baby? What, here? Now?" the guy said. "Really?"

"Yeah, like in a couple more minutes."

"Wow…yeah, I'll come back tomorrow," and he started to turn away.

"Who's at the door?" hollered Belinda.

"Just the mailman with something that needs to be signed for. He said he'll come back tomorrow."

Quickly, as another contraction was about to begin, Belinda said, "No! Wait, I know what it is, and I want it. I need it now."

The woman at the door called the mailman back. He returned, confused, and stuck his head inside. "What? I'm happy to come back tomorrow, you know."

Belinda pushed, and the baby's head began to show. The mailman's eyes bugged out as he stared, and Belinda's husband said, "It's the baby blanket that my wife's mother wrapped her in when she first came home from the hospital. We want it…but I'm busy…I can't sign now."

Finished pushing, Belinda glanced up and said, "Jeez, you're practically inside already. You wanna come in and watch? Then we'll sign, and you can be on your way."

"*Me?* Watch somebody have a baby? Oh, *hell* yes!" He put down his bag, his pad of receipts, and the package for Belinda, and he joined the crowd.

He actually missed about half an hour of work. The baby was born one or two contractions after he stepped all the way inside, but then he got the required signature and accepted a half glass of white wine and a hunk of barbecued ribs. He watched as the package was opened and the hand-knit blanket was admired and then put into the oven to warm.

Finally, he congratulated Belinda, shook hands all around, grinned from ear to ear, and gathered up his bag and receipt pad. Shaking his head, he munched on a brownie as he walked away, laughing.

Belinda looked up from her nursing baby and asked me, "Have you ever had the mailman drop in for a birth before?

That was an easy question to answer. I didn't even have to think about it.

"Nope."

That Tooth Has to Come Out

When she was five months pregnant, Jenna transferred to my care from an obstetrician. She smiled at me during her first prenatal visit, and the effect was shocking. One of her front teeth was missing. The fact that her husband, Ted, was a dentist and had done the original work on that tooth made it all the more bizarre.

But Jenna's whole obstetrical history was bizarre. She brought a copy of her prenatal chart from the doctor, and the missing tooth was just the most obvious element.

Her situation required me to take a ginormous leap of faith each time she came for a visit. She was anemic. Tiny with the body of a ballerina even before the pregnancy, she was now gaunt, having gained only three pounds. This meant she'd actually lost about twenty pounds of her own body weight. And her uterus measured very small for her dates.

Jenna politely but adamantly refused to follow any conventional advice, and for this reason her former obstetrician had refused to continue caring for her. She relied exclusively on the recommendations of Amapola, a traditional Mexican *curandera* with a New Age spiritual and nutritional twist. Jenna was certain Amapola's advice and treatments were responsible for her being on the verge of giving birth to her first child.

And she may have been right. It's hard to argue with success.

But it's also difficult to continue caring for a woman whose every action seems to be in defiance of conventional wisdom, and I knew I would be relying on continued support from my backup doctor throughout the remainder of Jenna's pregnancy.

* * *

After Dr. Jackson had provided me with backup for two years, his malpractice insurance carrier somehow got wind of the fact that he was working with a midwife who attended home births. We never learned how that information came to their attention, nor did we know who had blown the whistle – although Dr. Jackson has his suspicions. The insurance company informed him that, unless he severed all ties with Carole and me, they would terminate his coverage.

Joe Weick, an obstetrician who was married to a midwife, and his partner, Hank Streitfeld, whose wife had given birth to their second daughter at home with Carole's assistance, graciously agreed to back us up.

So it was to Joe that I turned, seeking reassurance about continuing to care for Jenna, because she fell off all the curves for Normal during her highly unusual pregnancy.

* * *

Twice I asked her to see Joe, and twice she agreed.

Twice Joe came to me afterward and said, "What, is she crazy?"

And twice we agreed I should continue caring for her in spite of all the warning bells: What if she bleeds? What if she's too weak to labor well? What if the baby is too small to thrive? What if her malnutrition has affected the baby's health?

We both knew she would continue putting her faith in Amapola, and we both knew she would have this baby at home, with or without me.

So I soldiered on.

Jenna had miscarried several pregnancies in her first trimester and had lost two babies after twenty weeks. After her last heartbreaking mid-trimester loss, she'd been unable to conceive for four years.

Now she had carried this present pregnancy almost into her third trimester. It was the first time she'd reached this landmark, and in spite of her hollow cheeks and sharp collarbones, she looked radiant.

"Both of those other times, since I was feeling the baby move, I was so sure I'd make it. But the first one stopped moving and we found out he'd died when we went in for an ultrasound, so I had to be induced. The other one I lost spontaneously, just woke up in a puddle of blood one morning, and the baby was born at home within an hour."

"And after that, you didn't conceive again?" I had asked.

"No, and then I turned forty and knew my time was running out, so I found Amapola."

"What did she do to help you get pregnant again?"

"She massaged me weekly, really deep massage through the muscles of my lower abdomen," Jenna said. "Some of it was very painful, but she was convinced my pelvic organs were out of alignment and stuck together, so she separated and rearranged them. At least, that's what she said she was doing. And after the soreness from the deep massaging went away, I did feel better.

"After a few months of that, when she felt things were in the right place and staying there between her visits, she began giving me injections into my uterus. Right through my belly."

"Injections of what?" The very idea made my toes curl.

"Xylocaine, actually. Can you believe it? The same stuff Ted uses to numb his dental patients. She injected huge amounts, and then she did the massage again, strong massage, working the Xylocaine deep into the muscle of my womb. It hurt terribly."

"I can imagine. So, then what? You got pregnant?"

"No, and Amapola was puzzled. So she checked my *chi* again, reread my *chakras*, and said the energy was still blocked somewhere. She asked about my teeth and I told her Ted had done an implant on one of my top front teeth.

"She said, 'That's it. That tooth has to come out. That's the problem.'"

"Ted, of course, was appalled," she said. "And insulted. 'There's nothing wrong with that tooth,' he said. 'It's perfect.'"

But Amapola was insistent, and Jenna consented. So all of Ted's careful work was destroyed, and Jenna was left with a gaping hole in her mouth.

"Can I at least make a temporary bridge so she doesn't have to go around looking like this?" Ted asked.

But Amapola said, "No, the space must be open to let the *chi* flow."

Two months later, Jenna became pregnant for the first time in four years.

As soon as the pregnancy was confirmed, Amapola told Jenna what she could and couldn't eat. "She put me on a diet of only leafy green vegetables with no seasonings or herbs other than those she specifically gave me. No protein. No fats. No bread or sugar or salt. Just vegetables, so I've been shopping in Chinatown, eating green things I can't even pronounce. I eat a lot of very bland soup."

All I could think was…wow, no wonder she'd lost so much weight. Amapola occasionally allowed her to have some plain rice or a banana, but otherwise, Jenna ate only vegetable broth and stewed or steamed vegetables.

All. The. Time.

And she steadily became thinner, more tired, and more anemic.

And I steadily became more and more concerned.

Four weeks before her due date, she looked to be no more than five or six months pregnant, just a little belly bump. The rest of her was skin and bones. I hoped the baby was taking what she needed from her mother, because Jenna was certainly being depleted. In spite of her luminous eyes, her obvious joy, and her quiet composure, she was wasting away before my eyes.

Ted and I had a few quiet conversations in which we shared our concerns, but Jenna listened only to Amapola, and we couldn't force her to eat.

I saw her more frequently than usual in order to monitor her weight and the growth of her belly, but eventually Jenna refused to step on the scale any more.

"Amapola told me that my weight, which is just an arbitrary number on the scale, isn't important."

"But, Jenna, you're actually losing weight, and you can't afford to lose any more." It felt as though I was caring for a woman in a refugee camp, and I was really worried about her.

"Amapola says the diet will keep the baby small without compromising her brain growth," Jenna said. "And she says it will make my uterine muscles strong so I'll have a quick, efficient labor. Most of all, she says I shouldn't weigh myself any more, because it's only causing everyone to be stressed, and it's very important that I avoid stress."

Okay, then. No more weighing.

But each time I saw her, I wanted to feed her a rare steak and a baked potato with lots of butter. And cheesecake. And maybe a milkshake while she was waiting for the steak to be ready.

The following week, Jenna said, "Amapola says it's a little girl who will weigh just over five pounds and she'll be artistically gifted and very, very bright."

I hoped I didn't sound sarcastic when I asked, "Does she say when the baby will be born?"

"Yes. She'll come early in the afternoon, two weeks before my due date. Amapola will be there, too, of course. So I guess we should prepare for sometime next week."

Oh, boy. At last I would meet this woman who was making me lose sleep. A woman I was prepared to distrust. A woman I thought I might not like very much, perhaps not at all. A woman I suspect must be autocratic, bossy, and maybe more than a little crazy.

But then something released within me.

It felt like I opened my chest and allowed my heart to bloom as I heard myself say, "Jenna, would you like Amapola to catch your baby?"

"Oh! I never dreamed...Oh, yes! I'll ask her tonight." Her eyes glistened with unshed tears.

The more I thought about my spontaneous offer, the more it felt right, and the more relaxed I felt. I didn't need to be needed. I wasn't needed. I wasn't really in charge here, and I realized I never had been.

At many births, actually, I wasn't truly needed. Oh, sure, I made decisions and women followed my advice and I offered suggestions and I eased the birth process. But most of the time things would have worked out even if I hadn't been around. Usually I sat on my hands and watched labor unfold normally.

The art of midwifery is knowing when to stand and act, but mostly when to sit and wait.

But Jenna called me at home that night and said Amapola had declined the offer to catch her baby. She hadn't given a reason, just quietly said, "Oh, no thank you." Jenna sounded a little disappointed, and I couldn't blame her. To even be asked to attend a birth is an honor, but to be invited to participate in the process makes the majority of people glow with pride and eagerness.

Two weeks before her due date, Jenna's labor began at 10:00 am, right after her weekly yoga class ended. When I arrived at the house, Amapola opened the door, and I was surprised: she looked no different from a hundred other Mexican *abuelas* I'd encountered over the years. Nothing to set her apart as a spiritual healer who was light years beyond your average Berkeley alternative therapist. She would have looked entirely normal patting out corn tortillas by hand before putting them on the *comal*, or buying *chile ristras* at the *bodega*, or shopping at the central *mercado* and putting her vegetables into a little string bag.

She looked ordinary – except for her eyes.

Her eyes looked as if they'd seen things and traveled places and gained knowledge that the rest of us would never have an opportunity to share. Her eyes looked as if they were already focused beyond time and space. Her eyes were locked on something that felt far beyond my scope of reality.

As Amapola had predicted, labor was hard and fast. Amapola spent her time inserting thin acupuncture needles into Jenna's toes, ears, and, oddly, the tip of her nose. I whispered encouragement, stroked Jenna's thighs, and massaged her perineum. Ted confined himself to supporting Jenna's body, stroking her hair, and just loving her, leaving the rest to Amapola and me.

And a delicate little girl weighing almost six pounds was born in the early afternoon, again just as Amapola had predicted. She cried immediately and looked entirely healthy. Ted cut the umbilical cord, dressed the baby, wrapped her in layers of oven-warm blankets, and handed her back to Jenna.

"We're naming her Poppy," said Jenna, and Amapola's eyes grew misty, for *amapola* means poppy in Spanish. Wiping her eyes, she said, "I'll go fix some soup for everyone."

Later in the kitchen, I sat down to do charting. Soon Amapola placed a bowl of steaming soup before me, and she carried two bowls into the bedroom for Ted and Jenna. I looked into the bowl. Pale green water with some long unrecognizable stringy green stems floating around, and a few slivers of, I think, maybe celery. I took a spoonful. It tasted like hot water in which two lettuce leaves had briefly simmered. No salt. No flavor. No texture. Just…nothing.

From the bedroom, I heard Jenna say, "How much longer do I have to eat this soup?"

"Oh, you don't like it? Okay, you can eat whatever you want now, Miss Jenna."

Ted said, "Yes! Yes, yes, yes! What do you want, Jenna? A bloody steak? Zachary's deep-dish pizza? Spaghetti and garlic bread? A chicken burrito with guacamole, salsa, and sour cream?"

"Mmm, that might be too much too soon. Maybe salmon and some broccoli?"

"Done."

Amapola died six months later of cancer. A month before her

death, she told Jenna she had known she was terminally ill for more than a year. While she would very much have liked to be the one to catch Jenna's daughter, she wanted the baby born into the hands of a healthy woman.

I wished we had known. I'm sure all of us would have tried to change her mind. She probably still would have refused, but I would have liked to honor her.

Spontaneous Midwife

I caught Reva's first baby at home, and it was a joyous affair, with three other women from her Orthodox Jewish community also present. As I had attended two of those women at their own home births, Reva's birth felt very much like a reunion.

In my admittedly very limited experience, Orthodox Jewish men often played minor roles during their wives' labors and the birth of their babies. I didn't really know why, but I suspected they considered childbirth to be "women's business." At the births I attended in their tight community, that's just the way it was.

After the birth of her son, Reva became a strong advocate for home birth. She thought it was the only option worth considering and felt sorry for women choosing to have their babies with doctors in the hospital.

"It's not for everyone, Reva," I tried to tell her, but she was really on a soapbox.

Her neighbor, expecting her first baby in about three months, planned a hospital birth with a doctor, and I suspect Reva gave her no peace. It's all she talked about when she came to me for a Pap smear a few months later.

"She's *meshuga*, just crazy. I mean, if she has to have it in the hospital, which I think is ridiculous, at least she should have a midwife, not a doctor. I keep giving her your number, pushing it into her hand, sticking it on her refrigerator with one of the magnets, but like I said, she's crazy, so stubborn, and she won't pay attention to me."

"Jeez, Reva, maybe leave her alone. You're probably driving her nuts."

"But I really like her. I care about her. I want what's best for her. Oy vey, I'm having a very hard time with this."

"I can see that. But maybe you ought to back off. Otherwise, you might damage the friendship."

"You're right. You're probably right. Maybe."

I heard nothing more for several months. Then Reva called, wild with excitement. "I have to tell you what happened with my neighbor. Only I don't want to tell you on the phone. Can you come for coffee sometime this week?"

Oh, what midwife doesn't love a good birth story?

When I arrived at her house a few days later, she said, "Purim was last week, and look, I still have some *Hamantaschen* left over." On the table was a gold-rimmed plate mounded with triangular cookies with jam in the center.

"What's Purim?" I asked, and she explained that it's a long and complicated story that ends with the defeat of Haman, the enemy of the Jews during the time of Esther.

"The cookies represent Haman's triangular hat," she said, "and we eat them in celebration of his downfall.

Okay, then. They were delicious.

"So, what's your neighbor's story?" I asked, reaching for a third cookie.

"Oh, it was fantastic," Reva said, hugging herself and grinning. "Ron – that's Jolie's husband. You know, Jolie, my neighbor who was having her baby in the hospital?"

"Yeah, the one you wouldn't leave alone."

She gave me a look but went on with her story. "Anyway, he rang our doorbell about 9:00 pm last Monday. And he said, 'Jolie went into the bathroom after dinner.' He thought she might be in early labor because she was acting a little weird.

"Then he said, 'Now she's been there for two hours, and she's making funny noises.'"

"Oh, boy," I said.

"Yeah, and she wouldn't talk to him. And she'd locked the door."

"Oh, boy," I repeated.

"Exactly. So Ron said, since I'd had a baby not too long ago, would I come over and maybe try to talk to her, get her to unlock the door, at least. So I went over with him, and as soon as I walked into the house, *vey iz mir*, I could hear her making those sounds I made right before Binyomin was born. I told Ron to get Avi, my husband, and tell him to bring his toolbox.

"Avi got the door off the hinges pretty fast, and there was Jolie, crouching on the floor in the corner, leaning against the bathtub. We could already see the baby's dark hair between her legs. Avi left, of course. It wasn't proper for him to see Jolie like that. But Ron went right over to her, even though there was blood and everything was wet between her legs.

"And oh, Peggy! I caught her baby! I did it, I really did it! And I loved it. I want to do it again and again. Do you think I could be a midwife someday? We're going to move to Israel in a couple of years, and I know the orthodox women there aren't always treated nice by hospital doctors. Sometimes not even by the old *bubbes* who still do some home births."

So the woman who insisted she wanted a doctor to deliver her baby in the hospital had instead been delivered at home by her neighbor. And indeed, Reva got her wish. She and Avi moved to Israel two years later, where he went to rabbinical school, and she began midwifery training.

I felt as though, unintentionally, I'd passed the torch on to a new generation.

The Scent of Peppermint

I stood in the doorway of the waiting room and called, "Fay?"

My new client stood up. So did the tall, thin man beside her, and together they came toward the exam room. A heavy smell of peppermint followed them down the hallway as I walked behind them.

About thirty-five years old and pregnant with her first baby, Fay had doubtless been a redhead in her youth. More strawberry blond now than actual red, her hair had probably faded with the passing years, but her skin remained fair and covered with freckles.

Other members of her Christian Science congregation had referred Fay and Greg, her husband, to me, so I wasn't surprised when she refused routine blood work. My experience working with women of this faith has been that they would do any test I insisted on "for your own professional security." In other words, they didn't want their refusal to comply with some aspect of care to get *me* in any trouble or to jeopardize my license – or my relationship with my backup doctors or the hospital.

But otherwise, except for my assistance at the home births of their babies, they really wanted nothing at all.

With the door of the exam room closed for privacy, the smell of peppermint became stronger. When Fay undressed for a physical exam, the source of the smell was obvious. A layer of 4x4 gauze squares about an inch thick covered an area on her upper right shoulder, and the minty smell coming from it made my eyes water.

I didn't know for sure what I was dealing with, but I began to have my suspicions.

I performed all the routine components of the exam, studiously ignoring the elephant in the room till the very end.

I said, "Fay, your dates seem accurate, so you're baby is due in about three months, and everything seems normal. I don't have a problem with your declining to have lab work done, but may I take a look at what the bandage on your back is covering?"

They could not have been more polite, more circumspect, more serene as they gently declined my request.

"Fay has always had a lot of freckles and moles, especially on her back," Greg said. "One began to look different about eight months ago, but it's improved significantly with the help of our practitioner. We aren't interested in a medical diagnosis, so there really isn't a reason for anyone else to see it."

"It started to smell strange as it began to change with the help of our prayers," explained Fay. "We don't want to offend anyone, so we're using peppermint oil to cover the odor."

I nodded.

I was nearly sure, especially given her red hair and fair skin, that she had a large malignant melanoma. Perhaps it had already metastasized. Perhaps by this time, even if she were to consent to surgery, a bad prognosis awaited her.

And she didn't want to hear it.

An ongoing systemic disease process is usually a reason to refuse a home birth to a woman. In fact, it's most likely a reason to turn her over to the care of a doctor. But this was a Christian Science couple. They would no more permit a doctor to deal with her "situation" in a standard medical way than they would permit me to.

So I was stuck between protocols and the reality of the situation.

"I'm comfortable continuing your care," I said, after a few moments of thought, "if you'll consent to a visit with Joe Weick, my backup doctor. If he okays a home birth for you, then we're good to go."

They looked at each other briefly, and a barely discernible nod passed between them. "If that's what you need to feel protected, legally, then of course we'd be happy to see your doctor."

Fay and Greg saw Joe a few days later. As they had done with me, they politely declined to allow him to see beneath the bandage.

I met with him at the end of office hours that day, and he said, "Very nice couple, and you know, I'm as sure as you are that it's a malignant melanoma under that bulky dressing. But they are clear in their priorities, and no matter what happens, they'll never sue either one of us. Go ahead and deliver her at home. Whatever happens, at least they'll have shared a good birth experience."

"I was hoping you'd say that. Have you had many Christian Science women in your own practice?"

"No. They all come to you! But my wife's aunt was one. She lived till she was ninety-four and then died of congestive heart failure."

"Wow, good for her," I said.

"No! It was crazy. A little Lasix every day, and she could have gone on another five years."

"But..." and then I saw he was laughing.

"Yeah, they're just different, aren't they?" he said. "And generally, they live long and healthy lives."

So I continued caring for Fay, and except for the ache in my heart and the increasingly overpowering scent of the peppermint oil, she progressed to her due date without incident.

When I arrived to attend her birth, I met Mrs. McCracken, the practitioner they'd been working with for what was, by then, more than a year. Occasionally she read spiritual guidance passages aloud, but mostly Fay labored quietly with Greg at her side, whispering into her ear.

I had an opportunity to talk with Mrs. McCracken during a lull when neither of us seemed to be needed, and, admitting my ignorance of most aspects of the faith, I asked how they dealt with such conditions as diabetes...or cancer.

"Well, while we have some awareness of those words, we don't use them in our practice. We focus on balance and faith and the intention of the body to heal itself when something is amiss."

I was flummoxed. "So, if someone has diabetes...uh, do you ever give insulin? I mean, what happens to them?"

"Oh, it varies. Some get better. Some decide to take insulin. And some die. But it's all right, no matter what they choose. As long as it's their full and informed choice, we're accepting of all outcomes."

Okay, then.

I wasn't sure I understood the reasoning behind these decisions based on faith any better than I had at the beginning of my career, but I was in no position to judge.

After ten hours of normal labor, Fay gave birth to a seven-pound daughter, and they named her Margaret.

I saw Fay for the last time at the six-week post-partum checkup, and she seemed fine, except for that clinging smell of mint.

I didn't expect to learn what the future held for Fay, Greg, and their daughter, but I was wrong. I became midwife to Helen, another woman from their church, and she told me that Fay had died. I wasn't surprised, but out of respect for her beliefs and her friendship with Greg, I didn't ask any details...just expressed my sorrow for Greg's loss of both his wife and the mother of his child.

After Helen's baby was born, she invited me to come for hot chocolate one afternoon to see Greg and Fay's little girl...and during that visit, Greg talked with surprising openness about Fay's final months of life.

Everything had seemed normal for the baby's first six or seven months. Mrs. McCracken continued to visit. She regularly changed the dressing on Fay's shoulder, prayed, and shared scriptural passages with them. The baby thrived, and Fay and Greg were happy.

"Then," he said, "Fay began to tire more easily. She always took care of Margaret, but she wasn't keeping up with the housework, and sometimes she didn't go shopping for more than a week. I got a little testy with her a few times, and I regret it deeply, now. I just didn't understand what was happening, not really, until one day a few weeks before Margaret's first birthday.

"What happened then?" I asked, but part of me really didn't want to know.

"Fay was feeding Margaret in her highchair. I was doing paperwork in the living room when I heard Fay call my name. That was the last time I heard her voice, because when I looked at her, she didn't say anything. She just stared at me, and...I don't know...it was as if I could sense her trying to tell me something. Something like, 'You're going to have to manage on your own now.' Then she walked to the couch, lay down, and closed her eyes. I thought she was napping. She'd been doing a lot of that, but when her arm fell off the couch and just dangled, I knew something wasn't right. I went over and called her name. She opened her eyes briefly, and I think she was looking at me, but she didn't answer – and within fifteen minutes, she was unconscious. Three days later, she passed over."

Fortunately for Greg and his daughter, the story had a happy ending. Helen introduced Greg to a woman whose husband had died in an auto accident, and they eventually married. So Margaret grew up with her father, two older siblings, and a new mother who made it her life's work to love and care for all of them.

But I've never since felt the same about the smell of peppermint.

Unexpected

For home births, we midwives of the era asked couples to have at least one additional person at the birth, a person we called The Housemother. Women usually chose a woman, most often a woman who had experienced birth herself. The Housemother's job was to provide relief for the partner, if necessary, to keep the midwives fed and watered, go shopping, handle the phone, do laundry, tidy up after the birth, and stay at least four hours afterwards to watch over the new family. We also anticipated that, should a hospital transport be necessary, the Housemother would be the one to drive the car.

Barbara and Hank chose David to be their Housemother, a gay friend of Barbara's from her college days, and they could not have chosen better. A tall, slender man with a composed demeanor, David was a poet, an architect – and a born *doula*. One could say he was intuitively in touch with his feminine side.

Far more than just a Housemother, David was Barbara's primary support person.

Barbara's first labor was arduous, spanning three days and two sleepless nights. During the first night, she slept off and on, but when she was awake and on her feet, it was David who accompanied her as she wandered around their Berkeley Craftsman house in the Elmwood district. He stopped when she did, and he let her hang from his shoulders during contractions, taking on himself most of her pregnant weight as he rubbed her back, whispered to her – and smiled. That's what I remember most: David's quiet, calm smile.

I glanced at Hank. Here was another guy assuming the primary role of labor support, and I wondered how Hank felt about it. He caught my look and said, "It's fine, it's fine. This is why we asked David. I'm kind of high-strung, pretty intense a lot of the time. Both of us sensed David would be better at this job than I would. And we were right."

During the second night, Barbara couldn't tolerate lying down during the contractions, and it was too tiring to jump to her feet when each one began. So she stayed upright. David put some bluesy saxophone music on the CD player, then took Barbara in his arms…

…and he danced with her.

All night long.

The rest of us, perhaps six in all, sprawled around the room as if it were a flophouse, dozing off and on, sometimes sleeping soundly for an hour or more. Every time I opened my eyes, they were still dancing and David was still smiling as he stroked Barbara's back and arms. Sometimes he kissed her forehead. Sometimes he hummed and sometimes he whispered in her ear.

Barbara appeared to be asleep…but her feet were still moving to the quiet, sensual music, the sleepy sounds I imagined would come from a smoky, nearly empty New Orleans nightclub around four in the morning. Most of all, the two of them reminded me of a pair of exhausted dancers in one of those contests held during the Twenties, marathons that went on until the last couple standing was declared the winner and took home all the prize money.

At dawn of the third day, Barbara's labor finally began to cooperate. It never went quickly, it never got easier, and pushing took forever, but eventually a healthy baby boy was born. David watched from about twenty feet away, leaning with his back against a wall. His eyes twinkled, his smile broadened, and then he went into a spare room and took a long nap.

* * *

We all expected Barbara's second birth to be quick, a piece of cake by comparison. But it was not to be. Although it was half the length of her first birth, thirty-six hours is still a very long time to birth a second child. Again David was her rock. He didn't seem to need words to be effective. His presence, his touch, his rhythm, and perhaps most of all, his relaxed smile were all Barbara needed. At last a second son was born.

When it was time for me to leave, David carried some gear to my car. Before I climbed behind the wheel, I looked at this compassionate man and said, "David, you're welcome to attend all future births with me. I seldom say this to a guy, but you're a natural."

He smiled and patted my shoulder. I don't remember the sound of his voice. I can't recall anything he ever said during those long, long hours we spent together.

Just his smile.

* * *

So when Barbara became pregnant for a third time, everyone expected a labor similar to her first two. Long, hard, slow, and tiring.

A few days before her due date, Hank called early on a Sunday morning to say labor had just begun. It was merely a heads-up call to let me know the baby might be born sometime that day, but more likely on Monday or Tuesday.

Less than an hour later, he called again and sounded panicked. "Barb's acting really weird, and she insists the baby's coming right now. I'm sure she's wrong. I mean, she *must* be wrong, right? But I dunno, she's just so...so *weird*. Maybe you could come over and calm her down, because, I dunno, she's really acting crazy."

Well.

Starting with me in my nightgown, I dressed, loaded my car, and arrived at their house twelve minutes after Hank's call.

Still, I missed the birth.

When I arrived, Barbara was sprawled diagonally on a very messy bed, clutching a baby girl to her chest.

The baby, although slathered in meconium, appeared to be fine. Oddly, she had a stack of perhaps fifteen receiving blankets, fresh-from-the-dryer, pristine clean and still perfectly folded into tidy rectangles, piled on top of her. Most of all, she resembled a puddle of dark and viscous maple syrup beneath a stack of fluffy pancakes.

Barbara looked shell-shocked from what she later described as "a very violent labor," but she soon calmed down and just stared at the baby. "A girl," she whispered over and over. "It's a girl. We really have a girl."

Hank, however...

Hank was far from calm. Naked except for a brown terrycloth bathrobe flapping wide open, he paced from one end of the room to the other, shaking his hands as if to air dry them and muttering to himself. He barely acknowledged my arrival.

As they'd both been expecting another two-day affair, they hadn't called David yet, and oh, how I yearned for his calm presence in the midst of all the chaos.

I quickly checked Barbara, wiped the baby clean, and put a little elf cap on her sticky head. Then I dealt with the placenta and the cord, wrapped the baby properly in the top two blankets from the stack, and settled her back in her mother's arms.

Hank had stopped muttering, but he kept pacing.

"Hank, tie your bathrobe," said Barbara.

"Not yet. Not yet. Soon. Yeah. Probably soon," and off he went to the other end of the room.

I helped Barbara to the bathroom, and she showered while I changed the bed sheets. Finally settled in a clean bed and propped up with pillows, she nursed her daughter.

Hank, stopped, tied his bathrobe, and stood looking at Barbara as a slow smile spread across his face. "It's a girl, huh? It's really a girl? Wow."

I just had to ask. I had to. "So, what was the deal with the stack of blankets on top of the baby?"

Hank looked sheepish. "I'll go make breakfast," he said, and headed toward the kitchen.

Barbara laughed, then turned to me. She said they were both caught completely off guard by the ferocious speed of the birth, which had lasted less than an hour. Apparently, the baby flew out in a gush of meconium while Barb was still on her feet.

"Hank caught her before she hit the floor," Barbara said, "and then he pushed me onto the bed, threw the baby onto my chest, and started pacing.

"I yelled at him, 'Blankets! Get the baby blankets!'"

Hank had apparently stopped pacing exactly long enough to retrieve the entire neat stack of receiving blankets. He ran back to Barbara and laid the blankets, still perfectly folded, on top of the baby. Then he resumed his pacing, bathrobe swinging wide with each turn he made. That's when I arrived.

I had missed it, and it's just too bad David missed it, too.

Not Quite DIY

Amanda's first birth had been speedy by anyone's standards, about ninety minutes from her first suspicion that labor might be starting to the baby's head crowning.

I could tell I needed to hurry when her husband, Rob, called me, because of the sounds Amanda was making in the background.

I arrived in time to catch that little boy, but just barely.

So when Amanda became pregnant with her second baby a few years later, I talked to both her and her husband about the possibility that, although I would of course hurry, they might be managing this birth on their own.

I handed Rob a copy of the booklet Emergency Childbirth, and we reviewed it together. I coached him about trying to control the speed of a baby who seems intent on rocketing into the world. I brought a life-sized floppy doll that I used when I taught childbirth classes, and together we did a mock birth. I talked to him about supporting the perineum, especially if it blanched of color. I showed him how to keep the baby's head flexed to ensure that it doesn't extend too soon or too quickly, which can sometimes cause tearing.

But knowing that those finer aspects of "controlling" a birth would probably either fly from his mind in the stress of the moment – or be irrelevant in an extremely rapid birth, one in which the baby has turned on her afterburners – I talked mostly about what to do immediately after the birth while they awaited my arrival.

I emphasized that absolutely nothing needs to be done to the cord or the placenta, and that above all, he shouldn't cut the umbilical cord. The placenta continues to function for several minutes after the birth. Babies born with extraordinary speed sometimes appear shell-shocked at birth. Their eyes might be wide open, their arms might be flung wide…but they look catatonic and they often don't start breathing right away.

Often, the mothers look the same. For good reason, both mother and baby can appear simply astounded, blown away by the violent nature of the experience they've just shared.

In those cases, the longer the placenta keeps doing it job, the better. It will continue to supply the baby with oxygenated blood until the baby's lungs take over, thus assisting the newborn in making her transition from womb to room.

I told Rob if the baby quickly cried and flailed around, great – but not to be surprised if her color remained blue and she remained quiet for a minute or two. In order for Rob to assist the placenta with its mission, I suggested he rub the baby with a flannel blanket…not roughly, but vigorously. Blowing into the face of the newborn was another option he could try, if he remembered. A blast of air on a baby's face will usually make her startle and gasp…and that gasp is the initiation of breathing.

But then I reassured Rob, who was looking perhaps a tad overwhelmed by all this information, that nine times out of ten, babies born quickly are absolutely fine, and all he'd need to do would be dry her off, keep her warm, and wait till I arrived.

As Amanda's due date approached, I was perpetually anxious, cancelling a date across the Bay Bridge in San Francisco for dinner with friends. At certain times of day, traffic can be a real bear, and I just didn't feel comfortable at the thought of being that far away. Also, I made sure my car was gassed up, and I stashed Amanda's chart and all my equipment in my locked car, ready for a quick getaway.

But I still missed it.

Although I left my house within two minutes of her call that "I think something is happening," the baby was lying on Amanda's belly when I arrived. Rob had covered his daughter with a couple of receiving blankets and put a little elf cap on her head.

Amanda was entirely calm, just cooing to the squirming baby, and the baby, pink and healthy looking, was nuzzling around, trying to find her mother's nipple.

But Rob.

At this birth, it was Rob who looked catatonic. He had apparently gone onto autopilot for the birth, and he'd done a terrific job – but he hadn't quite recovered from the experience by the time I arrived about ten minutes after the fact.

He stood rigidly upright in the middle of the room, gazing at his wife and newborn daughter. Then he turned his attention to his slightly bloody hands, holding them in front of him at waist level.

Finally he looked at me.

"Great job, Rob," I said.

"Yeah. I guess. Thanks. But I'm done here."

"What do you mean?"

"I don't do placentas."

Sari

I had delivered a few Indian women over the years, so when a man called and mentioned the name of a former patient, I wasn't suspicious… just surprised that he began the conversation by saying, "Please to come now and deliver baby."

More a command than a question. Odd. Decidedly odd.

"What's her name? Do I know her?"

"Her name, it is Anju. Vanni, she tell me your name is a midwife, so I call you to come now for baby."

"Anju, she's in labor? Where are you?"

"Yes, yes. In labor," and he gave me the name and address of a hotel on Shattuck Avenue in downtown Berkeley. "Please, madam, please to come now."

"Has she seen a doctor?"

"Yes, she sees doctor a few times. But now comes the baby."

"When is the baby due?" I'd never met this couple. Was the baby at term? "Is she nine months pregnant?"

"months, yes. Baby number two. You will come now."

Call me a risk-taker. Call me altruistic. Call me crazy. There would be a measure of truth in each of those labels.

I loaded my car and drove to the hotel, a six-story brick structure that looked seedy from the street and even seedier when I entered the lobby. A silent desk clerk pointed me down a hallway, and I navigated threadbare carpeting, dim lighting, and sticky stairs as I made my way to the third floor. The corridor smelled of cumin, cigarette smoke, dust, and mildew.

A thin man puffing a dark brown cigarette opened the door to my knock. He said nothing, took a step backward, and barely made eye contact.

The room's appearance gave me pause. Bare wooden floors, a small table and chair, a TV, and a microwave. Nothing more except for a sink and toilet in an alcove.

And a bed.

A single bare mattress on a metal frame, a pillow, and a cheap nylon quilt.

On the bed lay…well, it must have been Anju, although she never once spoke to me. Wearing a turquoise sari, she lay on her side, gripping the bars of the headboard with one hand and clutching her sari tightly around her hips with the other. Her long rope of a braid trailed off the edge of the bed, and she stared at the wall in front of her.

Young. Late teens, maybe early twenties. Beautiful, very thin, black eyes with long lashes, immobile.

Frightened?

"Anju?"

No answer.

"Anju, my name is Peggy. I'm a midwife, and…"

The man with the evasive eyes came close, exhaling acrid smoke into my face as he said, "No English. She knows why you are come."

I coughed. "Please put out your cigarette," I said. "It's bad for the baby."

He raised his eyebrows, then dropped the cigarette and ground it into the wooden floor with the toe of his pointed black shoe.

I turned my attention back to the rigid young woman and saw a small pile of wet towels on the floor beside the bed.

It was her second baby. Her bag of water had broken, and her contractions seemed to be very close together. As each pain began, she pressed her knees together, straightened her legs, and gripped the folds of her sari even more firmly. And she turned her face into the dingy pillow, probably to muffle any sounds that might otherwise have escaped.

It seemed the baby would soon be born, so I pulled the table close to the bed and set out a few of my things. She had no supplies of her own in preparation for this birth. No suction bulb, no pile of absorbent Chux, no stack of clean baby blankets or clothing, no bowl for the afterbirth. Nothing.

Also, no sister or mother or auntie to hold her hand and wipe the sweat from her brow. No woman friend to coo into her ear, reassuring her that it would be over soon and all would be well.

Just this cold and distant man who sat on a wooden chair fifteen feet away, drinking chai from a chipped mug and toying with his pack of cigarettes.

I touched Anju's thigh and spoke. Although I knew she couldn't understand my words, I hoped she would sense the meaning behind them: that I was here to help her, not to hurt her. "Anju, the baby is coming fast. May I move your sari?" and I began to slide the silky fabric toward her waist.

Her response was to pull her sari back down and wrap it even more tightly around her body. I stopped, but I'd gotten a glimpse beneath the layers of fabric. She still wore her underpants, and smears of bloody mucus stained her thighs.

"How old is her other baby?" I asked the surly man.

"Almost two. He is in India with grandmother. So Anju can work in restaurant."

"And this baby? Will she keep it with her?"

"No. No, no. It go to India, too. Maybe two, three weeks. She work. Send money home for baby."

I had no words. The knowledge that I was about to deliver a baby that would be separated from its mother and sent to a distant continent in a few short weeks stunned me. Would she ever see either baby again? And who was this man to her? A husband? I doubted it. From her extreme modesty, her obvious fear, and her total silence, I began to suspect the pregnancy had resulted from an act of violence.

So I just sat there on the edge of the bed. I put my hand on her arm. Now and then I gave her tense fingers a squeeze. I wiped her hair off her face and gave her sips of water. I talked to her the same way I talked to other women in labor, saying the same words, hoping the sound of my voice, my tone, my calmness, would make her less fearful – less fearful at least of me, if not of the hawk-nosed man who just stared out the gray and fly-specked window.

I didn't try to move her sari again. I didn't touch her legs or her thighs. I didn't try to remove her underpants. And most of all, I didn't try to spread her legs. I wanted to avoid anything that might make the birth seem as traumatic as I suspected the conception had probably been.

Soon she grunted, and I saw the involuntary curl of the belly that signifies pushing. She rolled onto her other side, facing away from me.

"Anju, I'm going to touch you," and I slid my hand from her shoulders, down her back, and over her buttocks. She didn't recoil, so I kept my hand there, right under the curve of her bottom, and soon I felt it bulge as the baby's head descended.

All I did was apply counter-pressure as the baby emerged. His body emerged into her underpants and was completely born there, even though Anju's knees were clenched and her legs were straight. It was as if she was doing everything in her power to keep from giving birth – but nature will not be denied.

The baby cried. I pulled her sari up from behind, slid the baby out one leg of her panties…and a few minutes later, the placenta followed. Anju allowed me to rub her belly to help her uterus contract. I used the towels on the floor to soak up the small amount of blood, and I took a quick peek to assure myself that she hadn't torn.

I turned to the impassive man. "Do you have blankets for the baby? Towels? Something for the blood?"

He stood, went into the bathroom, returned with two small thin towels, and handed them to me. Not a word did he speak.

I dried the baby off with a towel and placed him in his mother's arms. She held him close, covering him with a fold of her sari, but she barely glanced at him. I put the other towel between her legs, inside her panties. Then I covered both her and her baby with the quilt.

I stayed almost two hours. As I prepared to leave, the man said, "How much?"

I named a price, and he peeled a small stack of hundred dollar bills from a wad in his pocket, then handed me the money. I had a strong sense he would have paid any amount I'd asked with no complaint.

Anju met my eyes only once, just as I was about to leave. Her stoic expression didn't change, but she looked directly at me and held my gaze for perhaps five seconds. Was there a message in her eyes? Was it thanks? Hate? A plea for help? An acknowledgment of hopelessness? An admission of her powerlessness?

I'll never know.

Driving home, I felt as though I'd attended a birth in a Third World country. I also felt dirty, like I'd participated in something evil. I passed the Berkeley police department and considered stopping and filing a report. But what would I say? What was my complaint? A woman who couldn't speak English and seemed fearful? A man who said he was her husband but didn't appear to love her? I had no proof of rape. I'd seen no signs of physical abuse. The baby was healthy. Would they even have bothered to make a visit?

I kept driving, figuring I'd get more information when I returned for a postpartum visit. Perhaps without the focus so totally on the impending birth, I could glean more knowledge.

When I knocked on the hotel room door the next day, no one answered. I turned the knob, and of course the room was bare. The monosyllabic desk clerk shrugged when I asked for the identification of the couple who'd been there the previous day. He turned the register book toward me...and it appeared the room had been unoccupied for more than two weeks.

I called Vanni to see if she knew where Anju lived, but she denied knowing anyone by that name.

Five years after I delivered Anju's baby, a scandal involving Lakireddy Bali Reddy's human trafficking, restaurant, and real estate empire in Berkeley made headlines after a seventeen-year-old victim of his crimes died from a carbon monoxide leak in one of his cheap apartment buildings.

As nearly everyone in Oakland and Berkeley did, I followed the case closely. Although Lakireddy himself was not the man with Anju that day, I was convinced he must have been part of Lakireddy's organization and that Anju was a victim of his criminal activity. She was probably "employed" in one of his many Berkeley Indian restaurants and doubtless had been taken advantage of sexually as well.

* * *

In light of the information that later surfaced as a result of the investigation, I regret not stopping at the police station after Anju's birth. I regret allowing a full day to pass before returning to the hotel. Maybe the man feared that, indeed, I *might* go to the police, so perhaps he had taken Anju and her baby away as soon as I left – but maybe not.

I don't know if it would have made a difference. At that time, neither I nor anyone had reason to suspect any such person as Lakireddy and his widespread criminal ring existed, but still: I knew something evil had happened to Anju.

If I had stopped at the police station, might my tale have initiated the investigation that subsequently brought a wicked man to justice? Could I have eliminated years from Lakireddy's reign of power? Might I have saved countless women and young girls from lives of hard work, forced sex, and abuse?

I'll never know. And I live with those unanswered questions.

For information on the now infamous case, check this link:

http://sfpublicpress.org/news/2012-02/how-an-infamous-berkeley-human-trafficking-case-fueled-reform

Ken and Barbie

I met Ken and Barbie in a local coffee shop where they came to interview me for a possible home birth.

Really. Ken and Barbie.

And here's the thing: they looked very much like those eleven-inch dolls idolized by millions of little girls. Cute. Blonde. Slim. Smiling. This version of Barbie now sitting in front of me wore jeweled sandals instead of impossibly high heels, and she was eating a croissant. She had flipped up hair and wore lots of mascara. Ken was ruggedly handsome.

I'm sure they had long ago tired of all the jokes that must have been directed at them, so I said nothing.

"Our other kids were born in the hospital, and it was okay. But my sister just had her fourth baby at home with a midwife, and two women in our church have recently had home births, so it just got me to thinking," said Barbie.

"How many children do you have?"

"Four. So this'll be number five."

Big families are a little unusual in the Bay Area, at least among my client population. Then I recalled the word "church" in her comments, so I figured they were probably Mormon, Roman Catholic, or maybe evangelical Christians, couples who tend to "have as many babies as God chooses to bless us with."

As we talked, they decided on a home birth, but I think their minds were really made up before we even met.

Barbie was always immaculately groomed, and so were her children. She sometimes brought all four of them to her prenatal visits, and they were some of the most well-behaved kids I'd ever met.

The three oldest, ages eight, six, and four, generally stayed in the waiting room, reading quietly or playing with toys, while Barbie came back to the exam room. She kept the two-year-old with her, and he sat beside her on the exam table, his enormous blue eyes taking in everything.

Ken came to a few of the visits. I must have mentioned something about how busy they were going to be with five children under the age of eight. Barbie grinned and said, "Oh, I just love babies. I'll take as many as God sees fit to give us," and she hugged her little boy and ruffled his hair.

Ken said, "Well, God sure had a lot to do with it, but so did your sister, honey."

I was confused. Her sister? What could her sister possibly have done to contribute to the coming of their fifth child?

"Well, now..." Barbie was smiling at her husband. No, not just smiling. She was batting her eyelashes and tucking her chin into her shoulder, looking at him sideways. My lord, she was actually flirting!

"I warned you, didn't I?" Ken said. "I warned you not to pick up that baby."

Man, I was confused. "What are you guys talking about?"

Barbie looked coy. She giggled, and her eyes sparkled below her thick black eyelashes. "When my sister's baby was just a few days old," she said, "we all went over to visit. And oh, I do love little bitty babies, especially when their heads are still all floppy and they smell so good, you know, down in their necks. And those little kitty noises they make, like mewing..."

"And I saw that look in her eyes," said Ken. "I saw it, and I just knew what would happen if she picked up that baby and cuddled it. That's all it takes with her, just picking up somebody's newborn, and bam! She gets pregnant again."

"Well, honey, that's not *all* it takes."

"Pretty much, it is. I told you. When I saw you headed for that baby, I told you. I said, 'Barbie, do *not* pick up that baby. Do Not Pick Up That Baby.' But I blinked, and there you were, snuggling it and sniffing it and cooing to it and lovin' on it."

"Oh, he's right, he's right. But I do love babies. God just meant for us to have a houseful, I think."

I love babies, too. A lot. But having a baby every two years into the foreseeable future was a concept I found difficult to grasp.

Barbie's labor began sometime in the middle of the night. Their four-bedroom ranch house in the suburbs was still dark when I arrived before dawn, but about an hour later, I heard little footsteps running along the hallway. The two youngest children tumbled onto the bed, and half an hour later, the other two joined us.

And the dog. A pretty big dog.

Four kids, a dog, a husband, and a midwife shared a king-size bed with a woman who was happily approaching late labor. Barbie's cheerfulness, patience, and good humor were boundless. She didn't even object when the youngest rolled on top of her in the middle of a strong contraction.

Then she glanced at the bedside clock and said, "Oh, look at the time! It's a school day." Speaking to the eight-year-old, the only girl, she said, "Kacey, please change the baby's diaper, dress him, fix him a bottle, and turn on cartoons for him. Then get cereal for yourself and the others, okay?"

Having received her marching orders, Kacey left with the toddler. Ken shouted after her as she headed down the hallway, "And honey, when you've done that, let me know, and I'll come lead morning prayers."

"And Gabe, you're a big boy, right? You're six. Whooo, wait a sec. Here comes a big one…" and she sailed right through another contraction with only a little heavy breathing. "Okay, where was I?"

"I'm a big boy," said Gabe.

"Right," said Barbie. "And big boys know how to make peanut butter sandwiches, don't they? So will you please make three sandwiches? One for yourself, one for your big sister, and one for your little brother. Get dressed, then help your brother get dressed. When you're ready, Dad will take y'all next door, and you can wait for the school bus there."

My head was spinning. I could learn something from this woman. My kids, ages eight and ten, had rarely made their own school lunches. I was thinking Barbie's kids would probably be doing the family laundry by the time they were in third grade.

To the four-year-old, she said, "Be sure to brush your teeth, and help Davy brush his. Dad will take you over next door, too, and you can go on to preschool with your friend."

All this was accomplished in the space of three contractions. Four kids had their assignments, and four kids obeyed without any fuss.

The baby was born about an hour later with an equal lack of fuss.

"Oh, look, honey," said Barbie. "It's a girl. Oh, Kacey will be so happy to have a baby sister."

"Yeah, and like you're not going to be thrilled to have another one yourself, another girl to put in pink, with big old bows in her hair," said Ken.

Barbie ducked her head and smiled. Flirting again, only ten minutes after giving birth.

Two years later, Ken called me. "Well, now Barbie's gone and done it again. She's been lovin' on her friends' newborns, even though I keep telling her not to."

Seven months passed, and I delivered her fourth son. Two more girls came along later. A grand total of eight.

Barbie really did love babies. And she was really a flirt.

The Door's Open

It was Shirley's first baby. As a nurse in the Neonatal Intensive Care Unit in a local hospital, she worked day in and day out with sick, premature, or compromised babies. At her job, no normal, healthy, full-term babies ever came under her care. Quite literally, she had never had exposure to normal labor, normal birth, or healthy babies.

Yet still, she trusted.

As things transpired, she was blessed (or cursed, depending on your perspective) with a super fast Slam Bam kind of labor. She called early on to let me know things had started, but she called back about three hours later to say she was sorry, maybe she was wrong, not really sure, but perhaps I ought to come.

I stayed on the phone to listen to her during a contraction…and oh, yes, I left right away.

Shirley lived way, way, way up at the top of the Berkeley hills, and I had a good half-hour drive ahead of me. I might have done a California Curtsey at a few stop signs, and I might have treated a few red lights as if they were mere stop signs. Let's just say that I hustled and leave it at that. I mean, where's a cop when you really need one? I could definitely have used a few sirens and flashing lights on that trip.

I parked in front of her house and hurried up a series of wide stone steps to the front door. I must have made quite a racket with all my gear because as I approached the door, I heard Shirley shout, "The door's open, and I'm pushing."

Yep. She sure was.

I didn't even need to check her to recognize all the signs of imminent birth. She wore nothing but a crop top, and she stood in front of a huge stone fireplace, leaning forward with her hands on the wall above the mantle. As she pushed, she pressed into the chimney wall, shoving against it as if she were trying to push it over and destroy the entire wall.

Gary, Shirley's husband, never having experienced childbirth before but knowing these things usually take a good bit of time, came wandering in from the dining room, loading film into a camera (remember those days?).

I said, "Gary!" and he looked up, startled. I told him to open my blue tackle box and get out a few things. He did, but I had no time to get them organized. Bare-handed, I caught the baby about eight minutes after I arrived.

Shirley turned around, lowered herself to the hearthrug, and took the howling baby from my wet hands.

Gary looked as shell-shocked as if a tornado had just taken the roof off their house. "That's *it?*" he asked. "I mean...*what? It's all over? I thought it was supposed to take hours and hours."

"Well, yes," I said. "It usually does, but, as you can see, not always."

They had plans to bury the placenta in the backyard and then plant an apricot tree over the site a few months later.

Usually, people hang out with the baby, recovering from the birth, and celebrating with family. Maybe pop the cork on a bottle of champagne, have some food, admire the baby...

They generally double seal the afterbirth in plastic and then bury it a few days later.

But Gary was still a little spooked by the speed of the process, and he had energy to work off. He clearly wanted that placenta in the ground as soon as possible. The baby was less than half an hour old when he picked up the bowl and disappeared through the door to the garage.

An hour passed. Maybe longer.

"What's taking him so long?" asked Shirley.

"I was wondering the same thing," I muttered. I mean, during his wife's brief labor, he'd been focused on loading the camera, and now he was missing the first few hours of his son's life.

I went into the garage, then over to the door to the backyard...and I swear, he had dug a hole large enough to entomb half of my VW Beetle.

"Gary, jeez, what on earth are you doing?"

Shirley had followed me. Baby in her arms, she stood open-mouthed, then said, "Dude, what the hell?"

By this time, he was standing thigh deep in the hole and rapidly expanding it in depth and circumference with each giant shovelful.

106

"We live way up here in the hills," he explained, "and there are lots of wild animals around..."

"Not too many grizzlies, though," Shirley whispered to me.

"...and I want to be sure I bury the placenta deep enough so they can't dig it up."

"I think you've got it covered," Shirley and I said at the same time.

An End – and a Beginning

Melanie was pregnant with her second child. When I took her history, she revealed that her first baby had died of crib death (SIDS) at the age of seven months. I expressed my sympathy, and we talked a bit about the experience, the fact that it might have played a role in her marriage ending, how long it took to get over the loss, the acknowledgment that one never truly "gets over" the premature loss of a child.

And in reality, the loss of every child is premature. It's in opposition to the natural flow of life. Children simply aren't supposed to die before their parents. It feels as though the universe has turned upside-down and made a terrible, terrible mistake.

Five years had passed since her baby had died, she had remarried, and she wanted a home birth. It was my habit to make a home visit about four weeks before every woman's due date. I did this for many reasons: to check the accuracy of the woman's hand-drawn map in that pre-GPS era, to check that she had all her birth supplies, to become familiar with the layout of the house, to have a more leisurely visit on her turf, perhaps an opportunity to meet her partner and other children…stuff like that. It was always a relaxed visit, usually lasting more than an hour as we shared a cup of tea and talked about her birth plans, her hopes for how things would be handled.

Melanie's house was far up among the towering firs and eucalyptus in the Berkeley hills, and her quiet demeanor was reflected in the style of the house. Tattered Tibetan prayer flags in faded colors hung over the entryway, and wind chimes whispered somewhere among the trees. Inside, large brown and mauve pillows and folded futons constituted most of the furniture. Small, multi-paned windows in the diminutive fairy tale-like cottage let in minimal light on the thickly wooded slope, so the interior was muted and peaceful.

Melanie brewed intense Chinese tea in a small black cast iron teapot, and we sat talking for a while. Then she said, "I want to show you something." She was wearing a loose Indian print blouse and a long gauzy tiered skirt. She rose effortlessly to her feet, straight up and without using her hands – a subtle but powerful athletic feat I doubt I've been capable of since I was about ten – and she left the room.

I remained seated on my pile of cushions, sipping my tea as I waited for her return. When she came back, she had a photo album in her hands, and she sat beside me and opened it.

"This is Blossom, just a few minutes old," she said, showing me the first picture in the album, and I knew it was the baby who had died. She turned the pages slowly, and together we looked at pictures of Blossom smiling, Blossom being bathed in the kitchen sink, cuddled in a Snugli, lying on her belly surrounded by toys. Then Blossom could sit up…and she was eating a teething biscuit, damp crumbs all over her face. At the bottom of one page, Blossom was on all fours, clearly mastering crawling. She had a huge grin on her face.

I turned the page…and it was blank.

So were the rest of the pages.

I looked at Melanie, and my eyes filled with tears as I comprehended the enormity of what I was seeing. The blank pages stretched forever.

"And that was the end of Blossom," she said.

When I'd recovered a little, I shared with Melanie my eldest son's story of Spirit Babies, the story – or philosophy – that had comforted me when I lost a pregnancy. This boy of mine, twelve years old at the time, put his arm around my shoulder and told me that every woman has a host of potential babies circling over her head. If she becomes pregnant but loses the baby, its spirit goes back up into the circle, and it's always at the head of the line. So the next time she gets pregnant, she'll give birth to a Spirit Baby.[1]

"But if for some reason the woman doesn't have another baby," he continued, "the Spirit Baby is *beamed up* into the circle above another woman's head, and here's the really cool thing, Mom. All the other babies give it cuts, so it's always first in line."

Melanie was in tears. She reached out and held my hand to her cheek, then asked, "But where did he get that?"

"I haven't any idea," I said. "He said he was a Spirit Baby himself – which was true as I'd lost a pregnancy before conceiving him. He

---

[1] See Peggy Vincent's first book, *Baby Catcher: Chronicles of a Modern Midwife* for the complete story of Spirit Babies.

said it was just something he'd always known, and he was surprised that it was news to me."

"You have a wise child. Thank him for me."

* * *

Three weeks later, Melanie's husband, Ravi, called me. I heard an edge of anxiety in his voice as he whispered, "I wish you would come now, I really do. It's only been an hour, but I'd feel a lot better if you were here. She's not communicating much, and she's doing this weird kinda singing. Beautiful in a way, but just...weird. Mostly, though, I'm feeling totally out of my element here."

In the background I could hear Melanie's voice... and it *was* beautiful, just as Ravi had said. It had a transcendent and calming tone to it, and it reminded me of nothing so much as the deep and seemingly endless intonation of a Tibetan prayer bowl. They're also called singing bowls, and most are copper or brass. When you tap one with a felted mallet, it produces a soft gong that's prolonged almost indefinitely as you circle the rim with the mallet.

When I hear one, the effect on me is more a feeling than a sound. I can sense my heart, my whole chest and belly, vibrating to an otherworldly power...and that's how Melanie's humming was affecting me.

"I'll be right there," I said.

In fact, there were several hours remaining before she was ready to give birth. But if Ravi was feeling out of his element, Melanie had clearly found hers. She was wholly involved with the rhythms of her body and the sounds she was creating.

It would have felt like sacrilege to talk to her, to interrupt her state of concentration in any way, so I just listened to the baby's heartbeat and remained quiet. Ravi looked at me, a question in his glance, and I sensed he thought I ought to be *doing* something. I smiled, gave him a thumbs-up sign, and put a finger to my lips. He nodded, and together we sat, holding a vigil, trying to match our energy and state of being with the stillness of the mood Melanie had created.

She never really changed her demeanor. Usually when I'm with a woman in labor, I can make a rough guess what stage she's in by her appearance, her vocalizations, her behavior between and also during the contractions.

But not with Melanie. Nothing at all changed for two more hours. She had definitely achieved a trance-like state, and the humming never ceased. It didn't stop between the contractions, and it didn't change in tone or volume during them. Her eyes remained closed, and except for noticing her bare belly rise and tighten rhythmically, I had difficulty telling when she was having a contraction.

Then, still without opening her eyes, Melanie slid lower in the bed so she was reclining against a pile of pillows instead of sitting up cross-legged. I saw her belly tuck and curl as involuntary pushing began, and I slid some Chux behind her to protect the pillows. Not two minutes later, the bag of water bulged at the vaginal opening and then broke with an audible pop.

And still she hummed.

"Whoa," whispered Ravi.

I put a bath towel between Melanie's legs to soak up the puddle of clear amniotic fluid.

Melanie's eyes remained closed, but a small smile curled at the corners of her mouth. Her humming continued. She put her hand between her legs...and Ravi and I could see the baby's dark hair appear between Melanie's spread fingers.

I never touched her. I never touched the baby. I didn't speak, and neither did she. I kept my eyes wide open and watched – and I'm sure Ravi kept his open, too, probably wider even than mine – but Melanie's eyes were shut as she gently and slowly guided her baby from her body.

It wasn't something we'd discussed prior to the birth. It wasn't something she requested during the labor. It had just...happened. It felt as though it had been ordained, a mystery, a confluence of powers that made everything feel exactly right.

She lifted the baby girl onto her chest. Then at last she opened her eyes and looked at the child she'd just brought into the world.

"Hello, Fleur," she said. "You're our Spirit Baby, and we're so happy you chose us.

Backpedaling

Katherine's first labor was three hours, start to finish.

Her second was about ninety minutes.

When she became pregnant a third time, I was on Red Alert for the whole last month.

So was Bernie, Katherine's husband. He was so anxious that he was afraid to leave her alone long enough to go to the grocery store.

She told me one afternoon she'd walked to the mailbox about two blocks away to post a letter, "and when I turned around to head back home, I practically ran into Bernie. He'd *followed* me, for heaven's sake. I told him to leave off, dammit, cuz he's driving me crazy."

"I can't help it," Bernie said. "I feel like I should hang a peach basket between her legs in case this baby falls out while she's walking down the grocery store aisle."

I could definitely sympathize with him...and worse, I was obligated to teach a class in San Francisco two weeks before Katherine was due. I was decidedly nervous, anxious at the possibility of being stuck in traffic in the city and her having a slam-bam labor thirty to sixty minutes away, back in Berkeley. I was reluctant to cross that bridge into San Francisco, but I knew I must.

I half-considered having both of them come with me, but then I squashed that idea. After all, when babies come so fast that the birth is literally a catch by whomever is nearest at hand, things are usually just fine. Sometimes these babies are stunned at birth, a little breathless and wide-eyed at the speed of their ejection, but they rarely need more than time, patience, and maybe some vigorous drying off to get them started.

Bernie, however, really wasn't at all keen on the idea of being alone for the birth. Because I knew it was a real possibility, I had a special meeting with him. I gave him a copy of *Emergency Childbirth* and a couple of pamphlets used as teaching aids by the fire department. And together, we did a dress rehearsal as I gave him a mini-class on How to Catch a Baby.

I emphasized several points: try to control the speed of the baby's exit with gentle counter pressure, put the baby directly onto Katherine's chest, dry her off and cover her to keep her warm, and don't mess with the cord or placenta. On the chance that this actually happened while I was in San Francisco, in which case it could take me as much as an hour to arrive, he had the option of calling 911 if he was worried about anything or if Katherine lost more than a cup or two of blood.

Even more importantly, I made sure he had the phone numbers of my assistants, as well as all the other midwives in the area.

I made it to the city to teach the class and back home with no problem. And no baby. Another week passed with me on tenterhooks, checking my pager and its batteries several times a day.

Finally, Bernie called and said, "She's really quiet and she's acting weird."

I probably didn't even let him finish his single sentence before heading for my car, which had been loaded for more than a week. They lived on the second floor of a large pale blue Victorian, just a little over a mile from my house.

When I entered through the front door, I saw Katherine at the far end of the house, in the kitchen. She wore black leotards, a black long-sleeved turtleneck knit top, and a dark green corduroy sleeveless maternity dress. And shoes. And her hair was perfectly combed.

It was a very different scenario from those that had greeted me with her two previous precipitous births. With her first baby, she'd been naked when I arrived, pacing frantically around the house while she hummed and moaned loudly. Second time, she was just getting out of the bathtub as I entered the bedroom, and she barely made it to the bed before the baby sailed out.

This time, she was quiet and composed, but she was vigorously scrubbing the kitchen counter.

I said, "So. This one is different, huh? How are you doing?"

She didn't even look at me. She just kept her eyes on the countertop as she said, "It's coming right now. I've just been holding off so you could get here."

"Where are the kids?" I asked.

Katherine didn't answer, just scrubbed harder.

Bernie said, "We sent them to our friends in the downstairs flat about fifteen minutes ago, as soon as we figured it was happening fast again."

It was then that I realized Katherine was standing on one leg. Her other foot was twisted around the opposite ankle, and she seemed to be squeezing her knees together. And she was scrubbing the same spot over and over and over, making tight little circles on the granite with a tiny piece of paper toweling.

She glanced at me, threw the paper toweling into the sink, kicked off her shoes, pulled the dress over her head, and ran to the bedroom. She made it almost to the bed before dropping to the floor, where she began pulling at her leotard. I was about to cut a hole in the crotch of the tight garment, but together we somehow managed to get it below her knees.

There were only a few contractions remaining, but with each one, Katherine dug in her heels and pushed herself away from me, backpedaling several feet with each one. Bernie and I followed behind her on all fours, with me dragging my meager package of clamps and gauze squares and suction bulb along in my wake.

She back-scrabbled herself, crab-like, right out the bedroom and back into the kitchen – and the baby was born three feet from where she'd been standing when I arrived.

The placenta arrived without fanfare two minutes later.

Bernie was accustomed to his wife's unusual births, so he didn't seem at all fazed by this latest speedy drama. Together, we pulled her tights all the way off, washed her off a bit, helped her to her feet, and settled her and the baby into the pristine bed.

No need to change the bed linens. A few swipes with a mop on the linoleum kitchen floor…and we were all cleaned up.

"Efficient," I said.

"Yup," he said.

Sisters

Sarita was planning a home birth with her second child...but a tree fell and did severe damage to the roof and the rear half of her house. Fortunately, no one was injured, but major repairs were necessary, and as her due date approached, it was clear a home birth was probably not going to be an option.

To repurpose Gertrude Stein's famous quote, *There was no there, there.*

When she discovered the workers using her clean stack of cloth baby diapers as rags, she caved in and registered with the hospital.

So when labor was underway, we headed to Kaiser Hospital in Oakland. They weren't as "visitor friendly" then as they are now, and the labor rooms were minuscule with very few amenities. A stainless steel toilet folded up beneath the sink, and there was no shower. The room was wide enough for a single hospital bed with maybe four feet of space beside it. And a single chair was wedged between the bed and the wall.

Therefore, because of the limited size and also because hospitals just love making arbitrary rules, they were pretty rigid about enforcing their Only One Visitor At A Time rule.

Sarita's husband and I took turns for a while, but it seemed ridiculous, so I just...stayed. Sarita was in heavy labor, and then she got stuck. She was close to full dilation, but the baby was high and she hadn't progressed in more than an hour.

The residents and doctors began to mutter about a Cesarean.

"Okay, girlfriend, you have to get out of that bed and on your feet," I said. "Squat, swing from the doorknobs, dance, do calisthenics, whatever. Just do not *stay* on your back in that bed one minute longer."

Groaning in protest, she hauled herself out of the bed and walked back and forth for the entire claustrophobic ten-foot length of the narrow room. With each contraction, she grabbed the shoulders of either her husband or me, swung her butt from side to side, and moaned loudly.

Something was definitely happening.

Then she squatted and gave a pretty convincing push, a push that ended with a long growl that brought a nurse in at a trot.

She looked at the husband. She looked at Sarita, hair stuck to her sweaty face, crouching on the floor...and then there I was, crouching on the floor with my bare hand between Sarita's legs. I could feel the baby's head begin to push against my palm.

"What? Who are *you?* Are you *sisters?*"

Sarita and I looked at each other. Fair-haired, fair-skinned, close to the same age, blue eyes...and in unison, we put our arms around each other's shoulders and shouted, "*Yes!*"

"Well, sister, get her off the floor and into the bed while I find the doctor," and she left.

I delivered the baby on the floor with the next contraction, but before the nurse returned with a doctor in tow, we managed to get Sarita back into the bed, clutching the screaming baby to her chest. I threw a thick flannel sheet on the floor to cover the water and blood.

"Well," said the doctor, "at least she didn't have the baby on the floor," and he delivered the afterbirth.

As the doctor was messing with charting, Sarita's husband turned to me and said, "Sisters, huh?"

"What?" said the doctor, turning around.

"Nothing. Just a private joke."

Changes

Late in 1983, my practice began to change.

Sandi had been my primary assistant at home births for four years, but in January 1984, she would be leaving to attend midwifery school herself at the Medical University of South Carolina in Charleston. She would be gone a full year.

And Joe Weick was putting pressure on Alta Bates to grant me – and by extension, additional midwives in the future – delivery privileges. Married to a midwife, Dr. Weick was a vocal advocate of midwifery practice. Eventually, when he sensed the other obstetricians aligning themselves in opposition, he initiated a lawsuit through the federal government, asserting "restraint of trade." Had this been carried forward, it would have meant the hospital and all of its affiliated physicians would no longer be able to collect Medicare payments.

His lawsuit didn't make him popular with the other obstetricians, but his efforts were producing grudging and hard-won results...and I knew sooner, rather than later, I would be able to deliver women who wanted a midwife, but who weren't comfortable with the idea of a home birth. Equally important to me would be my ability to continue caring for a home birth mom who, due to some problem, needed to be transferred to the hospital during labor. No longer would I need to step aside upon arrival at the hospital and turn these women over to an obstetrician.

I suspected that, once I could deliver women in the hospital, the number of women seeking my services would increase significantly. Plus, my time would be divided between births both at home and in the hospital. Conceivably, I would be expected to be in two places at once.

Clearly, I needed help. Another pair of hands during prenatal clinic hours and assistance at home births were obviously the first priorities.

Bonnie Bruce, a birth center and delivery room nurse with years of experience, was eager to help me, but she was obligated to work at the hospital four shifts a week. She wouldn't necessarily be able to come at a moment's notice, as Sandi had always managed to do. To replace Sandi, I would need at least one other person in addition to Bonnie.

Margaret Love neatly stepped into the gap. Her own three children had been born at home, all of them rapid and uncomplicated births. Her first two babies had been caught by a lay midwife, a term we used in that era when referring to midwives who learned their skills via the apprentice route, without attending midwifery school. They were unlicensed and operated under the radar, always figuratively looking over their shoulders, fearing prosecution. I gave them high marks for courage.

Carole, with Sandi assisting, had caught Margaret's third baby.

Margaret taught exercise classes to pregnant women as well as childbirth preparation classes. She'd also gone to several births as a coach, and the Midwifery Bug had definitely bitten her. Talking with Sandi after the birth of her third child, Margaret mentioned that she really wanted to become a midwife and was interested in an apprenticeship.

She wondered, Did Sandi know how she might find someone with whom to apprentice? Did she know of an opening in an existing practice?

Why, yes, as she herself would be leaving the Bay Area for a year, Sandi did indeed know of a possible opportunity!

All the local midwives gathered irregularly at someone's house. These meetings were open to anyone who wanted to come, and they provided a place where we could support each other through the struggles we all faced, share knowledge, and suggest solutions to common issues. Sandi invited Margaret to attend one of these meetings in order to introduce herself to all of us, but especially to me.

Margaret sat beside me, and we clicked. It just felt right. Even though Margaret wasn't a nurse and had had no formal medical or midwifery training, it was quickly clear to me that she had the heart and the soul of a midwife and was meant to become one.

The next week, I called her to help me at a birth. In the time remaining before Sandi's departure, she and I began teaching Margaret the basics of providing prenatal care. It was a steep learning curve for someone who had never even taken a blood pressure before, but Margaret jumped in with both feet – and she learned quickly.

Soon it was time to let her catch a baby herself. Liz, a woman who had already given birth multiple times, was the perfect candidate. She and Sam, her husband, lived in a sprawling housing complex for married university students in North Berkeley on San Pablo Avenue. Because they already had four children, they qualified for one of the few apartments with three bedrooms. But the rooms were small, and there was only one bathroom. With the clutter and noise created by so many young children, it was pretty crowded and chaotic.

Margaret and Sandi and I mostly sat on the couch with kids climbing over us and yammering to each other while we watched Liz, chewing gum vigorously, walk up and down the short hallway. It was impossible to tell when she was having a contraction and when she wasn't; nothing about her demeanor changed.

Then she didn't come back, and we realized she'd detoured into her bedroom, so we joined her. Along with Sam, the kids wandered in one by one and stood beside the bed. They looked only mildly curious, and I'm pretty sure the youngest two had no concrete idea what was about to happen.

Sandi opened the rolled towel holding a few sterile instruments, and she added a pack of 4x4 gauze squares, a suction bulb, and an umbilical cord clamp. Margaret sat beside Liz, and I crouched close by, whispering instructions in Margaret's ear.

Liz removed her big wad of gum and silently handed it to her eldest child. She pushed quietly maybe three times, and then there was a baby boy in Margaret's hands.

Margaret unwrapped a loop of umbilical cord from the baby's neck and handed her up to Liz's waiting arms. Sandi wiped her down and covered her with a warm flannel blanket that Joe retrieved from the oven. I talked Margaret through the delivery of the placenta, which came along effortlessly a few minutes later...and we were done.

Margaret looked at Sandi and me and laughed. "Gee," she said, "that was pretty cool."

We laughed, and I said, "Well, they're not all this simple," but Sandi and I knew how she felt. The thrill of catching your first baby is something you never forget. All births are special, each unique and wonderful in its own way, but I'm sure every midwife remembers her very first time with extra fondness.

By the time Sandi flew to South Carolina in January, Margaret had attended quite a few births with us, and Sandi was relieved that her absence wouldn't leave me in the lurch.

And then my hospital privileges were granted in February.

Of course those treasured and hard-won privileges came with a long list of requirements, prohibitions, hoops to jump through, and limitations to the scope of my practice, but I knew with time and patience – not one of my outstanding qualities when it comes to dealing with bureaucracies – most of these roadblocks would ease off. Eventually I would truly be able to offer a full range of options to pregnant women.

And, indeed, the number of women calling me for care rose sharply. I wondered how so many of them heard the news so quickly... surely the Berkeley grapevine isn't *that* efficient...but hear of it they did. I suspect that busy ward clerk in Labor and Delivery had something to do with it, too. I really should have put her on my payroll.

Margaret was getting a crash course in midwifery. There were times I was busy with someone giving birth in the hospital when a woman planning a home birth called to alert me that labor had started – so I sent Margaret on ahead to evaluate her status in advance of my arrival.

Then, in May, I got pregnant.

I was forty-one when I conceived my third child, and Jill and Colin, my older children, were ten and twelve. I was *really* going to need help, so we began looking for an *au pair*.

In addition to Bonnie and Margaret, I had a list of other women, mostly OB nurse friends of mine, on whom I could call when I needed help. Mijo Horwich, Kathy Heilig, and Faith Koch, among others, stepped up when need arose, and Kathy went on to become a midwife herself. Carole, her partner, Ming, and I covered for each other when necessary, and one of my midwifery school classmates, Sara Pitta, was also available.

There were definitely some chaotic nights when it seemed as though all of our clients near their due dates decided to go into labor at the same time. Sometimes as my VW chugged north or south on Interstate 80 at 3:00 am, I figured we midwives were probably the only people on the freeway. We were out on the road together, sending our assistants on ahead to another laboring woman or swapping midwives midway through a labor. At times like that, it felt like we were playing a game of Musical Chairs.

But somehow it all worked out.

And Margaret was gaining a ton of experience.

Urban Issues

Like all large metropolitan cities, Oakland and Berkeley have safe neighborhoods and not-so-safe neighborhoods. As a home birth midwife, I'd visited them all. Lawyers living in mansions in tony Alta Piedmont, and teenage moms on MediCal living in West Oakland in apartments with peeling stucco and rusted balcony railings. Artists in factory lofts in industrial areas, and leftover hippies in urban communes.

I was never assaulted nor even felt threatened during my nighttime forays into any of these neighborhoods, but when I knew I was in a sketchier part of town at night, I tried to walk down the middle of the street, and I whistled very loudly between my car and my destination.

Just in case.

Returning from a birth at 2:00 am one foggy night, however, my usually trusty VW Bug died in the middle of the intersection in a very rough Oakland neighborhood, and of course this happened years in advance of cell phones.

I left the emergency lights blinking and started walking down the middle of a narrow, pot-holed street with trash blowing in the gutter and no lights visible in any of the houses. It was very dark, and I admit my heart might have been pounding just a little.

As I walked carefully along the cracked street, dodging syringes and dog shit, I remembered something that had happened just a few weeks earlier. I had called Margaret to evaluate a laboring woman for me, and she was walking from her house to her car when some guy ran up from behind and pushed her over. He yelled a curse at her, grabbed her purse, and took off. Fortunately, other than a skinned knee, some scratches, and a case of jitters, Margaret wasn't hurt.

Then she remembered that a placenta was tucked in her purse. She'd intended to give it to Jamie Westdal, who taught sibling preparation classes, but she forgot to refrigerate it upon her return from a birth earlier that day.

"I wish I could be a fly on the wall when he opens that plastic bag," she said later, when she told me about the incident. "Whatever reaction he has, I really hope it includes a long siege of relentless projectile vomiting."

After that experience, she never left her house at night without a mug of scalding tea – or just plain boiling water – in her hand.

So I continued down the street with visions of lurking muggers on my mind.

Then I heard loud reggae music, and saw a house with lights blazing behind a sagging screen door. I stopped and stood about six steps below the door, just listening. And watching.

The distinctive smell of marijuana wafted out to greet me. Loud laughter followed. I noticed a broken light dangling from a wire above the front door. A big guy with dreads and a torn, red Bob Marley T-shirt came into my line of sight. Another guy with a shaved head covered in tattoos rose to meet him, and they shared a joint.

I took a deep breath. Darkness, gloom, and poverty stretched up and down the street. I was more than five miles from my house, so I didn't have a lot of choice. I walked up those last steps and tapped politely on the metal frame of the screen door.

Nothing. They couldn't hear me above the music.

I knocked louder, then rang the doorbell.

The guy with dreads turned and saw me, a forty-something pregnant woman, standing on his front stoop. His jaw dropped. He just stared.

"Who dat?" asked someone, probably Tattoo Guy.

"I...I don't know. Some lady..."

"Well, shit, man. What she want? Let her in."

So, through the screen, Dreads said, "Yeah?"

"My car died," I said, pointing down the street. "I think it's out of gas."

He pushed the screen door open a little bit and poked his head out. Way, way down at the intersection he could see my VW's flashing lights.

"I'd like to call my husband. Could I maybe...?"

"Yeah, sure, sure. You wanna come in and use the phone?"

Before I could answer, Tattoo Guy came to the door, stared at me, then said, "Damn, man, what you thinkin'? She a *white* lady. And she *pregnant!* She ain't gonna wanna come in here!"

126

Dreads and I looked at each other, and then he said, "We've got a cordless. You want me to bring it out to you?"

"No, actually, I'd rather come inside. Is that okay?"

"Yeah, yeah," and he opened the door all the way.

I walked into a room littered with empty pizza boxes, squashed beer cans, and racy magazines. Among the clutter on the coffee table were Zig-Zag roller papers, crumbled pot, a water pipe, and a Bic lighter.

Tattoo Guy stared at me as if I were ET, then picked up one of the magazines and tried unsuccessfully to cover all the drug paraphernalia. He looked sheepish (and it's not easy for a guy with an octopus tattooed on his head to look sheepish), gave a little incredulous bark of laughter, then beckoned me to follow him down a narrow hallway to the phone.

And so I called Rog, my husband, asked him to bring a gallon of gas, and gave him the address.

He showed up ten minutes later. When he came to the open door where I was standing, we exchanged a look, but neither of us spoke. I thanked Dreads and Tattoo Guy, and we left.

"What..." he began, when we were down on the sidewalk.

"Don't say anything," I whispered.

"But..."

"I'm fine. Let's just put the gas in my tank and go home."

And that's what we did.

Au Pair

My third baby was due in late February, and I didn't want my busy practice to interfere any more than necessary with my ability to nurse him on demand. I wanted a live-in *au pair* who would be ready and willing to grab the baby, hop in the car with me, and attend births at all times, night or day.

I put out some feelers to local organizations that arranged for *au pair* exchanges, but nothing promising came along, so I advertised in local papers. I did this a few months in advance of my due date, figuring it would be a good idea to introduce whomever we hired to the lifestyle of a family in which the mom was a busy midwife, and to the drama of birth itself before she began observing them regularly... with the additional responsibility of caring for a newborn.

One person answered my ad quickly: Àgi, a Swedish citizen born of Hungarian parents who had immigrated to Scandinavia when Àgi was five. She called, and it was obvious from our conversation that she was fluent in English. But best of all, she was already here in California, about an hour away in the town of Fremont.

When she came from Sweden, she had hoped to have "a California experience," but it hadn't worked out that way for her. The Fremont family lived in a residential area many miles from anything remotely interesting to a twenty-year-old European woman looking for adventure. There was no public transportation nearby, no subway, no tram, and the family wasn't interested in teaching her to drive or giving her access to one of their cars.

So when she finished with her *au pair* duties each day, she was stranded – and she was desperate for a change of scenery. For some stores, movie theaters, coffee shops, discos, proximity to the excitement of San Francisco.... Anything other than a suburban street lined with houses and nothing more than a swing set in the back yard for entertainment.

We scheduled an interview in early January. An hour before I expected her arrival, I happened to be looking out our living room window, and I saw a short, dark-haired woman wearing a blue dress walking down our street. I'd never seen her before. She was taking her time, looking from side to side, sort of checking everything out as if she were looking for a missing cat. Or a house number.

Besides her curiosity and the fact that her face was unfamiliar to me, I think it was her shoes that made me notice her. She was wearing high heels. Not stilettos, but definitely high heels...and we simply don't see women wearing dresses and high heels walking down our street. It's just not a Bay Area look. Not at all.

I wondered if it was Àgi, if perhaps she had arrived more than an hour early for our meeting. But the woman passed our house and kept walking down the street toward College Avenue a block away – a street where there are coffee shops, specialty cheese stores, clothing boutiques, a big toy store, a library, and much, much more. Also a BART (Bay Area Rapid Transit) station and a bus stop. Berkeley is five minutes from our house, and San Francisco is twenty minutes away by BART. Our neighborhood, including College Avenue, was – and remains – a sought-out destination for locals and tourists alike.

An hour later, the doorbell rang – and there stood the woman in heels and a blue dress. It turned out she had deliberately arrived ninety minutes early, but her purpose was to thoroughly check out our neighborhood. She didn't want to find herself again living in an area where nothing ever seemed to happen. Having quickly seen that College Avenue was a Happening Scene, she very much wanted to be our *au pair*.

It was settled quickly, and two weeks later she moved into a back bedroom just off our kitchen. She fit into the family with amazing ease, and just a week after her arrival she saw her first birth.

But we almost missed it.

Alice's first child, a boy, had been delivered by a Sufi midwife in Southern California. For years, Alice had been a devoted follower of Sufism, which is sometimes referred to as a sect of Islam. But when I asked her, Alice described it to me as "an inner mystical dimension of Islam, not separate from it in any way." The Sufi most people have heard of is Rumi, a well-known thirteenth century poet, mystic, and teacher.

When Alice's due date was just ten days away, her *mawla*, her spiritual Sufi leader, died – and she desperately wanted to attend his funeral service in Los Angeles.

She did her homework. She located her former midwife, who agreed to catch her baby should she go into labor before returning to Berkeley. She would be gone only two nights, so she packed very little in her carryon suitcase other than her birthing supplies and clothing for a newborn. Her husband, Charlie, stayed behind to care for their toddler during his wife's brief absence.

Sometimes, airlines refuse to allow pregnant women to board planes if they are "too close to delivery," but as Alice was carrying her baby mostly inside her belly instead of sticking way out in front, I didn't think it would be a problem.

So off she went.

Two days later, she returned before noon and called me to check in. She said, "On the return flight, I was having lots of cramping, and now I just noticed a tiny bit of bloody show. Maybe it'll start up for real pretty soon."

I didn't hear from her any more for the rest of the day and went to bed around 10:00 pm.

Àgi, who had been with us only about a week, came quietly to our bedroom door at 12:15 am and whispered, "Peggy?"

Instantly, I was wide awake, as I'd heard something between fear and awe in her voice. I sat bolt upright and said, "What? What?"

"The phone rang a few times..."

I glanced down and saw the extension beside my bed had become unplugged from the wall. Oh, lord...what's happened? I wondered.

"I've been hearing the phone ring for more than an hour, maybe four times, so I finally went in to listen to the message, and this man just said, 'It's Charlie again, and I can see the baby's head now...'"

"What the hell?" I cried. I looked at my pager, but it had no message in the window. Why hadn't Charlie paged me? "Get dressed," I said to Àgi. "You're coming with me. And hurry."

"What?" muttered my husband. I was usually really quiet when slipping off for a birth, but this night I was like a madwoman clattering and chattering around our bedroom.

"I'm leaving. Sorry. Go back to sleep."

I called Margaret and said only, "Come to Alice's," hung up, and then I pulled a purple sweatshirt over my nightgown. I slid my bare feet into clogs, met Àgi at our front door, handed her half my gear, and away we sped.

Fortunately Alice and Charlie lived only ten minutes away, but with no traffic on the quiet streets at that hour and with my sense of urgency, we probably made the trip in less than seven minutes.

Also fortunately, the front door was unlocked. We ran inside and heard nothing.

Upstairs, we entered the bedroom…and were met by a scene that Àgi will surely never forget. Her eyes grew almost as large as the baby's crowning head, and she stopped in her tracks.

Alice was on all fours with her bottom facing the bedroom door. Her long brown hair hung forward and coiled on the sheet below her. Charlie was sitting calmly beside her, hands folded in his lap. Alice was panting lightly, but really, everything was very quiet. Kind of mystical, actually.

I didn't have time for gloves. I put my hand on the baby's head and said to Àgi, "Open that tackle box, take out the towel-wrapped package, and unfold it without touching the things inside."

She pulled herself from her trance and laid the supplies beside me.

With the next contraction, I asked Alice to keep panting, if she could manage to keep herself from pushing. "Just try to breathe all the way through the contraction, Alice. Breathe, breathe, that's it,"…and she did.

At the end of that contraction, the baby crowned fully – the widest diameter of the head filled the vaginal opening. Very slowly, I slid her perineum ever so gently past the infant's head before the next contraction began. If a woman has self-control and can resist the powerful urge to push, delivering a baby between contractions is a good technique to help prevent the skin from tearing.

Alice laughed softly and looked back between her legs, but she couldn't see anything. So she put her hand down and felt her baby's chin and mouth and nose while she waited for the next contraction to begin.

The shoulders stuck briefly, but as Alice was already on all fours, my preferred maternal position for managing shoulder dystocia (stubborn shoulders, most often associated with big babies), it wasn't difficult to resolve the issue. I ended up delivering the posterior shoulder first, and the rest of the baby followed quickly, along with a flood of meconium-stained fluid.

The fluid that previously had puddled between Alice's knees was clear, which meant the baby had probably pooped the meconium when the head was already low in the vagina, so she hadn't aspirated any of the dark water.

She was tangled up in the umbilical cord, too – twice around the neck, then across her shoulder and once around her belly. By flipping her left and right, it wasn't difficult to unwrap her and give her a quick once over. Alice was still watching from her upside-down vantage point between her legs.

"Turn over, Alice, and I'll hand her to you." Usually I slide a baby forward to a mom who's on her hands and knees, but I didn't want to push her through the sea of meconium on the sheet.

The baby cried as Alice rolled over, and gathered her daughter into her arms.

And finally we could all take a breath. Àgi and I had left my house just seventeen minutes earlier. Margaret sailed into the bedroom and delivered the placenta while I stood up to stretch my stiff and aching back muscles. My own baby was due in just two weeks.

Then Alice began to bleed. Margaret grabbed her uterus, elevated it, and massaged it vigorously in an effort to encourage it to contract, and I began a thorough exam to see if she had lacerated her cervix or vagina.

Alice was uncomfortable with all this poking and prodding. She handed the infant off to Àgi, who wrapped her snuggly in a flannel blanket and sat close to the warmth of a small fireplace to keep the baby warm. She ate an apple as she swayed side to side, rocking the baby.

Finally the bleeding stopped. Alice looked at Àgi holding her baby, then she looked at Charlie. "Sophie?" she said.

"Or Michelle," said Charlie.

Alice looked back at Àgi. "Sophie or Michelle? You choose."

"Me?" squeaked Àgi. "You want me to name the baby?"

"Sure," said Charlie. "Sophie or Michelle. You can pick, cuz we like them both."

Àgi looked at the baby's face, then said, "She looks like a Sophie to me."

"Sophie it shall be, then," said Alice.

Turning to me, now that everything had been dealt with and

resolved, including the baby's name, Charlie said, "Wow, I'm really glad you made it."

"Charlie, I'm so sorry. The phone in my bedroom somehow became unplugged – maybe one of the cats, I don't know. But I didn't hear the downstairs phone ringing."

"Oh, that's okay. I thought you were just listening to my messages, deciding when it was time to come."

"*What?* No. No, no, no." I couldn't believe it! "Did you *really* think I'd just sit there listening to your messages and not pick up the phone to *talk* to you?"

"Well…I guess. I mean, everything was going along fine."

'Did you page me?"

"No."

"*Why?*"

"I didn't want to bother you. I figured the pager was for emergencies, and this didn't seem like an emergency."

I looked at Margaret, and she rolled her eyes.

I sighed. "Okay. Well, I finally got here. But…jeez, dude…" And I thought of the shoulder issue, the meconium, the cord entanglement, the bleeding…

"So, then…how did you decide to come?" he asked.

"I *didn't*. I wouldn't have even known you'd called if it weren't for Àgi here, our brand new *au pair*. She heard you say you could see the baby's head, and she came upstairs to waken me."

Àgi had awakened me at 12:15 AM, and the baby was born at 12:35.

A month later, Àgi told me she thought she might be pregnant… and she was right.

Skylar, my third and last baby, was born three weeks after Alice's birth.[2] From then on, Àgi, carrying Skylar in his straw Moses basket, and I went to nearly every birth together. When she was five months pregnant, a client of mine who had birthed what she swore was her last child gave Àgi her entire maternity wardrobe, so she looked very stylish during the remainder of her stay in the Bay Area.

By the time Àgi returned to Sweden in September to have her own

---

[2] For a detailed account of Peggy Vincent's home birth with Skylar, her third child, see Baby Catcher: Chronicles of a Modern Midwife (Scribner 2002).

baby, she knew a whole lot more about childbirth than your average first-time mom. Her son, Jesse, was born on the twentieth of October 1985.

Not Like Your Party

Dr. Brian Gideon's wife, Cathy, was pregnant with their third child, and so was I. Coincidentally, his wife and I shared the same due date.

Brian was one of the "good guys," the kind of obstetrician who respected his patients and tried to provide them with the best possible birth experience he could choreograph. He was equally respectful of the nurses, listened to their opinions, and appreciated the little things they could do to make his life easier.

He was always gracious, soft-spoken, and I can't recall ever seeing him really angry. When he was on call on the weekends, he nearly always brought in goodies for the OB nurses.

While everything progressed without a hitch for me, Cathy was diagnosed with a partial placenta previa in the early months of her pregnancy.

With ultrasound usage having become so frequent and widespread, the diagnosis of low-lying or partial previa has increased enormously. But in nearly all cases, by the end of the pregnancy the condition has resolved and presents no problem to a normal vaginal delivery.

Usually the fertilized egg comes wandering down the Fallopian tube and imbeds as soon as it lands on the soft, spongy cushion of endometrial tissue awaiting its arrival in the top half of the uterus, right where it's supposed to be...and the baby develops below it.

But in some cases, the fertilized egg wanders around a bit longer than is really necessary and chooses to embed somewhere in the lower half of the uterus. Then it begins to grow, and in growing, the edge of the developing placenta can appear on ultrasound to be encroaching on the cervix.

But here's the great thing, the saving grace of this situation: a growing placenta seeks the site of the best blood supply, the richest "food source," and that location is higher up in the uterus. So, if serial ultrasounds are done (as they frequently are, nowadays) to track the location of the placenta, it will show the placenta growing upward, away from the cervix and toward the top half of the uterus. It appears as if the placenta is wise enough to know that down there is not the best place to be hanging out, and it had better crawl its way higher up the uterine wall.

At the time of birth, the only evidence that might remain of this diagnosis is an umbilical cord insertion closer to the edge of the placenta as opposed to a central insertion, which is usually the case.

Dr. Gideon and I talked about this. We both knew the chances of Cathy's placental location continuing to be a problem were remote, but still, he was a little anxious, mildly concerned that it might progress to a real placenta previa.

In such a situation, if the worst happens, the placenta remains low in the uterus, spreading right over the top of the cervix. It's in front of the baby, and, if undiagnosed, it's a recipe for disaster. When the cervix begins to dilate, it exposes large and critical blood vessels in the placenta, which can bleed torrentially. This can rapidly cause the baby's death...and also the mother's, if surgery isn't done very, very quickly.

There is an old saying in obstetrics, which fortunately turns out to be true in the vast majority of cases: "The first time a woman with previa bleeds isn't a killer; it's a warning." After diagnosis of a total placenta previa, women are hospitalized so, should hemorrhaging begin, she can be operated on at once. If bleeding remains absent or minimal, she stays on bed rest long enough for the baby to achieve maturity, and then a Cesarean is performed.

"Remember that time you saved my ass?" he asked me during one of our conversations.

I could actually think of more than one time, because nurses are a patient's last line of defense against physicians' unwitting mistakes. But at the moment, I didn't know which "saving of his ass" he was referring to.

"Which one?"

He laughed and said, "Yeah, more than one, I know, I know. But I'm talking about the lady with the previa, the one you stopped me from maybe killing."

"Ah. That one..." and it all came back.

* * *

Years earlier, when I'd still been a nurse working in the hospital, he came onto the unit to introduce himself to one of his partner's patients. He hadn't yet met this woman, nor was he familiar with her history.

He spent a few minutes with her chart, and then said, "I see she's early, but she's got a little bleeding. Can you come with me while I examine her?"

I stopped in my tracks and stared at him. "You're going to examine her? Like, do a vaginal exam?"

He stopped, too, right in the middle of the hallway. "Yeah," he said, then paused. "Why are you looking at me like that?"

"I'm thinking perhaps you're very, very crazy," I said.

"What? Why?"

"She's got a previa."

Absolutely the last thing you want to do to a woman with a confirmed placenta previa is a vaginal exam. A finger probing up the cervical canal can poke directly into the placenta and provoke exactly the kind of bleeding you just never, ever want to see.

"No, no. That was with her first pregnancy, and she had a Cesarean, of course. But I don't see any reason why she shouldn't try for a vaginal birth this time."

"She's got a previa again, Brian."

"No."

"Yeah."

"No," but he narrowed his eyes and looked hard at me. "Really?"

"Really."

"No way."

"Way."

He turned on his heel, saying, "Just lemme go look at her chart again," and within half an hour, we were preparing the woman for her second Cesarean.

* * *

As my pregnancy continued to progress smoothly, Dr. Gideon's wife's partial previa condition resolved exactly as the vast majority of these cases usually do. With no further reasons for concern, he and his wife planned a hospital birth with Cathy being delivered by one of her husband's partners.

The months passed...and my third baby was born at home.

When Skylar was about a week old, I took him to the hospital to

139

introduce him to my friends who were working that day. Dr. Gideon happened to be there, too. He had brought the nurses a pound of Peet's Italian Roast and a bag of Noah's bagels with three kinds of *schmear*, and he was brewing a fresh pot of coffee for everyone when I walked into the room.

"Ah! You had him!" Brian said, grinning at me. "At home, right? Everything went okay?"

"Yeah, it was quite a party," I said. "What about your wife, has she delivered yet?

"Oh, yes, yes. I'll tell you about it later. Let's talk about you."

Having smoothly deflected the conversation, he excused himself a few minutes later and returned to the main desk while I ate a bagel with spicy roasted tomato *schmear* and shared details of my birth experience with my friends and former coworkers.

Then I went looking for Brian.

He saw me headed his way and began walking on a tangent so we met up in a private side corridor. "Your birth ended with a big party, huh?"

"Yeah, there was quite a crowd," I said. "But what about yours? Why so secretive?"

"Well," and he tilted his head back and smiled up at the ceiling. "It was quite a party for us, too. But probably very, very different from the one you had."

"How so?"

"Cathy shook me about 6:00 am. 'Wake up,' she said. 'It's time." She told me she'd been in labor for a few hours, but she'd let me sleep because she knew I'd been at the hospital most of the night. Then she headed downstairs.

"I was really tired. I was just lying there, getting ready to stand up, when she came back. She walked into the bedroom and just stood there and stared at me. She was wearing this big T-shirt of mine she'd been sleeping in. 'Get up. We need to get to the hospital, Brian,' she said, and she headed downstairs."

"She didn't change clothes?" I asked.

"Nope, and that should have been my first clue, but I was just so tired. So I went into the bathroom for a quick shower. Figured it'd help me wake up. I was all lathered up when the shower door opened. But there was no one there. At first I was confused, but then I looked down toward the floor.

"And there she was. Cathy. On all fours. Hair hanging in her face. All sweaty as hell. She looked up at me with fire in her eyes, and she snarled, "Now, Brian. *Now!*""

"Oh, my God. Do *not* tell me you…"

"Wait. Just wait," he said, and he was grinning. "So here's the thing. She'd taken off that T-shirt, so she's naked, see? I hop out of the shower, soaking wet, and sort of drag her through the house. I absolutely do *not* remember how we get downstairs, but we make it as far as the front door when she drops to the floor again, hollers really, really loud, just the one time…and that's where I delivered our son."

"You didn't. Really? You had a home birth? Awesome," I said.

"Well, since it was *not* what we'd planned, it didn't feel so awesome at the time.

Cathy was naked. The baby was naked. And I was naked, too. I mean, I still had shampoo in my ears."

I could easily visualize the scene, but then I had a thought. "Wait. You were trying to get her out the front door to take her to the hospital. But – you were both naked? What was your plan?"

"I hadn't gotten that far."

Do It Well

I was listening to the evening news as I prepared dinner.

"Damn!" I dropped the French chopping knife as my blood mingled with carrots and onions on the cutting board.

I held my finger under the faucet and watched red water flow down the drain. My daughter, Jill, looked at my hand and said, "Eeeuw, your finger guts are coming out." Indeed that's what it looked like as bubbles of finger fat overflowed the edges of a long gash down the side of my finger. She brought me a Band-Aid and I put it on tightly, but I couldn't stop the bleeding. This kind of stuff doesn't bother me at all, but really?

This was gross.

I knew I needed a few stitches. If it had been somewhere else on my body, I might actually have tried to sew it myself, but with just one hand, it was quite impossible.

So, while Àgi stayed home with the teenagers and the baby, my husband, Rog, drove me to the ER where a doctor stuffed my finger guts back inside and took five dainty stitches. A nurse applied an awkward and bulky dressing, gave me a tetanus shot…and dinner was late.

I had just finished nursing Skylar and putting him to bed when my phone rang. I smiled in spite of my throbbing finger.

Meghan O'Reilly. We'd been in a book group together, and after years as a single mom, she'd married Kevin, a big strong guy with luminous eyes and a gentle manner. This would be his first child. Meghan's two daughters, fifteen-year-old Aurora and ten-year-old Zephyr, were as excited as Kevin.

I took a couple of Excedrin and drove to a small, two-story house with many gables and lots of Victorian gingerbread dripping from the eaves.

I knew carrying my equipment would be uncomfortable with my wounded hand, but it was a pleasure making several trips to and from my car. The gardens leading to the house at the rear of the property begged to be admired in the dim light of a late summer evening.

Vegetables, herbs, and flowers in the sunniest parts of the yard, ferns and impatiens in the shade, baby's tears growing over damp stones, the pleasant sound of gravel crunching underfoot, a melodious wind chime in the distance, and a quiet fountain beneath a stone statue of a smiling Buddha…all contributed to a sense of peace and quiet.

Phil, a Zen priest, opened the door for me. I'd known him since I'd attended his wife's birth a few years earlier. His wise and humorous eyes peered at me from behind wire-rimmed glasses, and he helped me with my gear. He made no sound in his cloth slippers as he carried everything into a second-floor bedroom.

Then he noticed my big bandage. "Mmm, hurt hand?"

Economy in everything. Even words. Very Zen.

"Yeah, I cut my finger about five hours ago and needed some stitches."

"Can you deliver Meghan's baby like that?"

"I think so, but my assistant, Margaret, has done plenty of births, so she can manage if it's too awkward for me. But actually, Kevin plans to catch the baby himself."

"Ah. Well. Kevin. There may be a change of plans."

"Why?" I was perplexed. Kevin had been thrilled when Meghan and I had suggested he catch his daughter.

"He threw his back out, and he's been in bed the last two days."

"Oh dear," and then someone knocked on the door. "That's probably Margaret now," and Phil went back downstairs to let her in.

I turned around…and there was Kevin, flat on his back in bed. He turned his eyes toward me and fluttered his fingertips, but he didn't move his neck.

Not good. Not good at all.

"Oh, it's that bad?"

"Pretty bad, yes."

Wearing only a purple T-shirt, Meghan paced the room, her long black braid snaking down her back and swinging side to side with each ponderous step. A casual observer might have suspected she wasn't in labor at all, but her intensely focused gaze, her look of deliberate composure, and most of all a smear of bloody mucus on her upper thigh belied that first opinion. She was in active labor, more likely late labor. I didn't say anything, just smiled, checked the baby's heart rate, and felt the strength of her next contraction with my fingertips.

When that pain ended, she asked, "What happened to your hand?" but before I could answer, Margaret entered the room. On crutches.

"Whoa," said Meghan. "This is beginning to look like a casualty ward."

Margaret looked at me and asked, "What happened to you?"

"Kitchen incident. Stitches. What happened to you?"

I noticed a thick bandage on her knee that made my own look insignificant as she said, "Rheumatoid arthritis flare. Steroids, and the doctor drained it."

"Bet *that* was fun," I said, to which she replied, "Not."

"So," I said, looking around. "The gathering of the lame and frail." Between the three of us, Kevin, Margaret, and me, we had three legs, three hands, and two backs. Only Phil was truly able-bodied.

Then I noticed Aurora and Zephyr curled in a dim recess, a window seat overlooking the front garden.

Meghan resumed her pacing, Margaret and I set our supplies on the dresser, Kevin lay still and watched, Aurora braided Zephyr's hair…and Phil started to leave.

"Wait," I said. "Let me think a minute. Meghan's right – it really does feel like a hospital triage unit here. Can you stick around in case we need you? I mean, if it's okay with Meghan, of course."

Phil and I looked at her. She kept walking, didn't speak, just stuck both thumbs up.

I took that as a Yes.

Phil just nodded and smiled.

"And girls? Can you both help, if necessary? I mean *really* help, like hands-on kind of help?"

Zephyr blanched and frowned, but Aurora stood up and joined us in the middle of the room, eyes bright with anticipation of the unknown.

"Sure, I guess, but you'd have to tell me what to do."

"A lot depends on what position Meghan chooses when it's time for the birth…"

"Not the bed. Can't lie down," Meghan interrupted. "Just can't lie down, can't lie down, can't lie down at all."

"Okay, that pretty much settles it," I said to Margaret. "We're going to need some help."

"Yeah, cuz I can't get on the floor."

"I can get on the floor, but I can only use one hand."

"My back is fine, if she needs someone to hold her up," said Phil.

Kevin said, "I feel so useless. Useless and helpless…"

Meghan stopped pacing and stood at the bedside, facing him. "Just look at me. Don't stop looking at me. I could drown in your eyes."

Soon Meghan began holding her breath and grunting at the height of each contraction, and she leaned forward, resting her hands on the edge of the bed. A few contractions later, she motioned for Phil to stand behind her, and – locking her eyes on her husband's wide-eyed stare – settled into a semi-squat. Supported by Phil's arms, she reached over her head and clasped her hands behind his neck.

As Phil braced himself to take her weight, I said, "Aurora, I think you can catch your baby sister yourself. We'll help you."

"Really? Me?" she yelped. "Wow," and she ran to wash her hands. When she returned I motioned her to join me on the floor.

Meghan pushed in utter silence, and the baby's head began to show. Margaret managed the front part of the head while I applied counter-pressure to control the speed…and Aurora prepared herself for probably the most dramatic moment in her young life.

"Put your hand right where mine is," I said, and she did. "You have two hands. Use them both," then I put my one good hand on top of hers.

There wasn't a sound in the room. I glanced at Meghan. She and Kevin still stared at each other. It felt so powerful, so intimate. Holy, even.

Zephyr slid off the window seat and moved to the foot of the bed where she stood wide-eyed for the duration, one hand covering her mouth.

The baby's head came out easily, turned sideways, and she opened her eyes.

Aurora said, "Oh…" staring into her baby sister's face.

Meghan whispered, "I'm okay, I'm okay. I've got this."

Margaret and I removed our hands, and I began telling Aurora how to let the shoulders come one at a time, the top one first…but it wasn't necessary. In seconds, the whole wet, warm and wiggling baby squirmed in her big sister's hands.

Kevin's eyes filled with tears. "Oh. Oh, I had no idea…"

Phil peered over Meghan's shoulder, then looked at me with a Zen smile.

Meghan sighed and said, "Whoa, it felt so good to get her out."

Aurora, frozen in time with a squalling newborn in her hands, said, "What do I do now?"

We laughed, and I said, "Hand her up to your mom." She did. Then, holding her hands in front of her as if she's never seen them before, she went to the sink and washed them.

With our three good hands, Margaret and I dried the baby and wrapped her in oven-warm blankets. Then Meghan laid the newborn on her husband's chest while we dealt with the afterbirth and umbilical cord.

Sipping tea a while later, Kevin said, "Well, it's not the way we'd planned it, but I wouldn't change a thing."

"Me, either," said Meghan.

"Me, either," said Aurora.

Before leaving, Phil turned and said, "Kevin, I forget. How did you hurt your back?"

"Well, actually I was peeing...and I sneezed."

After we'd stopped laughing, Phil said, "Oh, Kevin, Kevin. How long have you been a Zen practitioner?"

"Gee, fifteen years, I guess. Why?"

"Fifteen years, and you still haven't absorbed the most important principle of all."

"What's that?" I asked.

"Do one thing at a time, and do it well."

More laughter...then I looked at my hand. Perhaps one day I, too, would learn to do just one thing at a time.

Chop vegetables or listen to the news.

Not both.

Just be very Zen about it.

It's Complicated

Her parents named her Esther, but at age sixteen, she changed her name to Hadassah, the Hebrew equivalent of Esther, when she joined a club at her high school for Jewish students interested in becoming more religious.

She met her future husband in that group, too. He was named David at birth, but he didn't think it sounded "Jewish enough," so he changed it to Ehud.

Hadassah and Ehud went to University of California at Davis, were married in an Orthodox ceremony midway through their sophomore year – and Hadassah gave birth to their first child, a girl, eleven months later in San Francisco, at Mt. Zion Hospital's birth center.

They named her Rivka, and when she was a few months old, they moved to Israel.

There, in Jerusalem, Hadassah finished her education. She deliberately nursed her daughter as much and as often as possible. She later told me that, as birth control wasn't permitted by their conservative Orthodox sect, breastfeeding frequently was her only option for delaying the return of her fertility. As she really wanted to finish school, she hoped to space her children at decent intervals.

Ehud attended a local *yeshiva* ("Torah school," Hadassah called it) to advance his study of the Torah and Talmud, and he did additional training to become a *shochet* and a *moyel* in order to supplement their income.

As a *shochet*, he was trained in ritual kosher slaughtering techniques, so he worked afternoons in a large butcher shop in central Jerusalem. And with his skill as a *moyel*, he was asked to perform the *bris*, the jubilant celebratory ritual at which Jewish baby boys are circumcised on their eighth day of life.

Curious, I asked Hadassah how much money a *moyel* charges, and she said, "They aren't supposed to charge anything, as it's a *mitzvah*, a blessing, to do the circumcision, but the family can offer any amount

149

they wish. And the *moyel* may accept it.

"Ehud has been paid anywhere from nothing more than a pan of potato *kugel* to $1000, but I guess it averages out around $400."

I learned all this backstory when she came to me pregnant for the second time.[3]

As her first birth had gone smoothly, she hoped to have a home birth this time. Rivka, her daughter, was three, so the dedicated amount of time she'd invested in breastfeeding while in Israel had worked out pretty well for her, in terms of child spacing.

Although Ehud worked as a butcher, he and Hadassah didn't eat meat. "It makes it so much easier to keep a kosher kitchen if you eliminate meat from your diet," she explained – but I already knew that. At least in Berkeley, vegetarianism was a pretty common practice among my more religiously-observant Jewish clients.

As she progressed into late pregnancy, Hadassah worried that she might go into labor on the Sabbath.

"Why would that be a problem?" I asked, and she said she really wanted her mother to attend the birth.

"So...?" I really didn't get it.

She explained that, unless it was an emergency, she wouldn't be able to use the telephone to call her mother, as it would be breaking one of the many religious laws that governed their lives.

"But...will you be able to call me?" I asked.

"Oh yes, because that would be an emergency. You understand? There's a difference between me needing a midwife at the birth, and just *wanting* my mother to come."

* * *

Then I remembered an incident about ten years earlier when I'd been a nurse at Alta Bates and had just admitted an Orthodox woman in active labor. After my patient had been with us for perhaps half an hour, the overhead operator made a very loud and insistent general

---

[3] My interactions with families who are members of any of the several branches of Orthodox Judaism have been minimal. While I don't profess to understand most of the philosophy or belief system that lies behind their lifestyle, I've grown to appreciate the strong sense of community that develops as a result of the practice of their faith. These recollections are mine alone and are not intended to represent any collective or universal "truth," as it applies to Orthodoxy.

announcement: "*A blue Ford sedan is parked in front of the hospital. The engine is running and the keys are in the ignition. Security is guarding the car. But it will be towed unless the owner appears immediately and moves the car to the parking garage.*"

My patient's husband muttered something, and I said, "What? Is that your car?"

"Yes, it's my car. But I can't move it."

"What? Why?"

"It's the Sabbath," he said.

"And...?"

"We are forbidden to light a fire on the Sabbath unless it's an emergency. Turning on the ignition of the car, which is considered "lighting a fire," to get my wife here to the hospital was permissible because it was an emergency. But I can't turn it off."

"I'm missing something here," I said. "Why couldn't you park the car properly and turn off the ignition?"

"Because that's considered to be "extinguishing a fire," he said. "That, too, is against the rules, so once I got Devorah here to the hospital, there was no longer any emergency."

I pondered the situation. And I wondered what purpose was served by a religious law requiring that someone leave a car running in a public area with the keys in the ignition – available for anyone to come along and steal. I had absolutely no knowledge, at that time, of the many rules that governed the lives of religious Jews, and consequently, this made no sense to me.

But it wasn't for me to question someone on the articles of his faith.

"Um, wow. But the car has to be moved. Would you like me to find someone to park it for you and then bring you the keys?"

"Oh yes, that would be a *mitzvah*. I wouldn't have asked you, but I will say Yes, if you offer."

"Well, I can't do it myself, because I'm responsible for your wife's care, but I'll find someone."

I called the operator first to let her know help was on the way and to call off the dogs so the car wouldn't be towed. Then I phoned the nursing station and explained the issue. Seconds later the ward clerk appeared in the labor room doorway and said, "I'll take care of it."

When she returned, she put the keys in the guy's hand and told him where she had parked his car. He thanked her profusely, referring to her as a *shabbos goy*.

"A what?" we both asked, and he explained that a *shabbos goy* is a friendly non-Jew who performs work on the Sabbath that *halaka*, Jewish religious law, enjoins an observant Jew from performing.

This was all a little complicated for me to work out rationally, so I forgot about it...but here I was, years later, coming face to face with a similar situation.

* * *

"So, if this baby comes on a Saturday, you can call me, but you can't call your mother, right?" She nodded, watching me...and I knew, I just knew, what she wanted me to say. "If that's the case, would you like me to call your mom?"

"Yes, oh yes," Hadassah said. "Please, yes. And thank you so much for understanding," and she wrote her mother's phone number on the top page of her chart.

Sure enough, her labor started on the Sabbath, and I dutifully called her mother, who arrived before me. She was sitting in the living room doing a puzzle with Rivka when I came through the door with Àgi and Skylar, now four months old, in tow.

When I greeted the grandmother and introduced myself, she sighed and rolled her eyes. "All this nonsense. Esther was a nice normal Jewish girl until she was sixteen, and then she went and got all religious on us. Changes her name, keeps kosher, follows *halaka*, and now her husband won't touch her."

"What do you mean?"

"Go back there. Just go back there and look at them. You'll see what I'm talking about. It's *meshuga*. Crazy, just crazy."

Margaret arrived minutes later, and we went back to the bedroom together. Àgi and Hadassah's mother stayed in the living room with Skylar and Rivka, who had instantly become totally absorbed with my smiling and wiggling son.

Hadassah was sitting partly upright on the large bed. In one hand she held a comb tightly in her fist, and in her other hand was a bottle of feminine deodorant spray. I had previously heard of such a product, but I couldn't recall actually having seen one before...and I found it kind of sad that she felt it necessary.

152

She was in good, strong labor, and alternately she brought each hand to her face, saying, "Ah-ha-heee, ah-ha-heee, ah-ha-heee," first to the comb, and then to the deodorant bottle.

Margaret stared at her, then whispered to me, "I remember hearing something about combs and acupressure points for pain relief, but I've never seen it before. But why isn't she holding her husband's hand?"

"I don't have any idea," I said, and we both looked at Ehud.

He sat on a very narrow single bed on the far side of the room, hands clasped between his knees, and he was rocking back and forth. He smiled at us and and raised his head in a greeting, then turned his gaze back toward his wife and resumed his subtle rocking.

Hadassah's labor progressed smoothly. As she moved into late labor and then began to feel like pushing, Ehud rose from his bed and stood beside her. He smiled, he offered kind words of encouragement, he seemed to understand and appreciate how hard she was working – but he stood three feet away and made no move to touch her. It was entirely up to Margaret and me to offer her sips of water, to smooth damp hair from her forehead, to stroke her back and remind her to keep her bottom relaxed.

The baby, a boy, was soon born. And still Ehud kept his distance. I placed the baby on his mother's chest, and she cooed to him, stroked his cheek, and smiled up at her husband.

He smiled back and said, "What a beautiful job you did, my pearl. And a son. Shall we call him Eitan?"

"I think Chaim is better," she said.

"Chaim it shall be."

The placenta came along in its own time, and I offered Ehud the opportunity to cut the cord. To my surprise, he recoiled and crossed his arms in front of his chest, blocking me from giving him the scissors. "No. No, no, no. I can't."

Okay, then.

Margaret and I dealt with the cord, dried the baby off, and began to wrap him in warm blankets. Hadassah said, "Could you give him a bath, please?"

"Now?" We almost never bathed a baby in its first hours of life.

"Yes, I know Ehud wants to hold him, but the baby must be clean."

Ah, I was beginning to understand. An Orthodox woman, I knew from my other admittedly few religious Jewish clients, is considered unclean until several days after her menstrual flow ceases...and as long as it takes following childbirth for her postpartum bleeding to stop. She then goes to the *mikvah*, a special deep pool of still water (no Jacuzzi jets here) used for ritual cleansing and purification. She may then resume sexual relations with her husband.

With the ritual *mikvah* immersion following menstruation by several days, her husband is permitted to return to her bed at pretty much the exact time of the month when she is most fertile...and this timing is a significant part of what accounts for the large number of children found in many Orthodox families.

In childbirth, when a couple is as deeply observant as Hadassah and Ehud were, from the moment a woman's water breaks or bloody show appears, she is considered unclean, and religious law prohibits her husband from having any contact with her.

The small single bed on the far side of the room was apparently where Ehud slept each month from the time Hadassah's menstrual period began until she returned from the *mikvah* about two weeks later, washed clean and purified once again.

So I realized that, as the baby was still wet with the blood, mucus, and amniotic fluid of the birth, Ehud probably considered the baby, as well as his wife, "unclean," even though Margaret had thoroughly dried him off.

Hadassah's mother was in the bedroom doorway. She followed me into the master bathroom and talked to me as I filled the sink with warm water. "See? See what I told you? He won't touch her, he hasn't touched her since a little drop of bloody mucus appeared early this morning, and now he won't even touch his own son until he's had a bath. Been 'cleansed.' An innocent baby that needs 'cleansing,' can you imagine? Oh, I hate seeing my only daughter caught up in this craziness, but will she listen? No, of course she won't."

"Well, I don't understand the rationale behind most of the religious laws either, but they seem like a really happy family, don't you think?"

"Yes, yes, they seem happy enough. But oh! I adore Rivka, and I want her to have more choices in her life, the chance to make up her own mind."

I squirted shampoo on the baby's thick dark hair, scrubbed it, then used a comb to be sure all traces of blood and vernix were removed. I washed in the folds of his neck, behind his ears, in the crease of his buttocks, his groin, between his fingers and toes…

By the time I finished, he was probably the cleanest infant in California.

While I helped Hadassah into the shower, Margaret and the baby's grandmother diapered and dressed him, wrapped him in flannel blankets…and finally his proud father gathered him into his arms.

As she had brought Skylar into the room for me to nurse a couple of times during the past few hours, Àgi had observed some of these interactions. On our way back home, she said, "I never saw that man kiss his wife or even touch her during her labor. Not once. Why is that, do you know?"

"It's complicated. It's a long story, and I'm probably not the right person to talk about it to you," I said, "but I'll give it a try." And I began to explain something to her that I didn't really begin to understand myself.

* * *

Again Hadassah nursed her baby for more than two years, and again she came to me for a home birth. This time, however, she carried the pregnancy beyond her due date. My agreement with my backup doctors was that I wouldn't attend a home birth if the woman was more than two weeks past her due date. As due dates are at best an educated guess, an additional day or two probably wouldn't have raised any eyebrows – provided all went well. But there were now two other midwives about to gain privileges at Alta Bates, and I didn't want to jeopardize any of our hard-won gains. If I chose to let a woman progress beyond two weeks post-date and delivered her at home, and if there were complications, I would come under an enormous, brightly-lit magnifying glass. Potentially there could be hell to pay, for me most certainly – but also for the other two midwives, simply by association.

So, when Hadassah was one week and six days beyond what we all agreed was a pretty accurate due date, we talked and came up with a plan that was based mostly on the fact that her cervix was super soft and already dilated to a stretchy three centimeters. Labor could start at any minute – or, conversely she might hang around for a few more days, which would put her beyond my limits for proceeding with a clear conscience.

Hadassah and Ehud understood my situation, and they really wanted a home birth, so together we formulated what we called Plan A.

She came into the hospital just before noon. A nurse strapped a fetal monitor onto her belly and conducted a non-stress test (NST). It's a test of fetal wellbeing: a reactive (good) test is one in which the baby moves three times in ten minutes, with a rise in the baby's heart rate with each kick. If she didn't pass the test, Plan B would be activated: Hadassah would stay in the hospital, and I would induce her.

But the baby aced the test. This simple test, however, would do nothing to encourage labor to begin, and the clock was ticking. So we moved ahead to the next step: I would rupture her bag of water. If the fluid was clear, we'd check the baby's condition for a short time, and then they would go home to await labor, which we hoped would begin that afternoon.

If meconium was present in the fluid, however, Plan B would go into effect: Hadassah would be induced, and her baby would be born in the hospital.

So, mentally crossing my fingers, I broke the amniotic sac.

Ta-da! Clear fluid! Over the next fifteen minutes, the monitor showed the baby's heart rate rising with several rapid kicks, and then we noticed that Hadassah had immediately begun having regular contractions.

Over the nurse's feeble – and mostly perfunctory – protests, I disconnected the fetal monitor, put a towel between Hadassah's legs, helped her into her underwear, and off we went.

It was not common for a woman pregnant with her third child, two weeks past her due date, in labor, and with her bag of water broken to leave the hospital and go home.

It fact, it was maybe even unheard of.

But that's what we did.

Ehud followed behind, taking care, now that water was leaking from her, not to touch his wife. He drove Hadassah back to their home, and I followed them in my own car, previously loaded with my birth supplies in the hope that things would unfold exactly as they had.

…and grateful once again for the fact that I had hospital privileges and was therefore able to choreograph what had just occurred. I smiled all the way down the freeway, feeling as though we'd really pulled off quite a coup.

I had called Margaret from the hospital, so she arrived just a few minutes after we pulled into the driveway. Hadassah's mother, with Rivka and Chaim at her side, met us at the front door, and she helped her daughter, now in very good labor, undress and pull on a loose T-shirt.

This time, Ehud's behavior didn't startle me, and Margaret and I worked together to assist Hadassah through what turned out to be a very efficient labor and birth. In the years since Chaim's birth, Hadassah's mother seemed to have made a degree of peace with her daughter's choice, so the tension and disapproval I'd felt during the previous birth were no longer present.

Two hours after we all arrived, another boy joined the family. This time, I didn't offer scissors to Ehud to cut the umbilical cord. And no one needed to ask me to bathe the baby before laying him in his father's arms.

I already knew what was required of me. I was a real *shabbos goy*.

But, still…it's complicated.

Just Not Ready

My midwifery practice was booming.

I worked loosely with Sandi as she was building her own practice, so when births piled up, we could cover for each other. Carole, too, although she lived nearly an hour away, was also willing to answer a call when the need arose. With a lot of forethought and planning, we found we could each actually take a vacation now and then.

But still, I was awfully busy. I had two kids going through puberty and a new baby who decided that ten months of age was just the perfect time to begin walking – only a month after he'd started crawling. Even with a live-in *au pair*, I had a lot on my plate.

I had a telephone at my bedside, of course, for answering nighttime calls, but the only phone downstairs was in the path of foot traffic from the front of our house to the back. When I returned home each day, there were usually several messages on the answering machine for me, each requiring a return phone call.

My oldest children really never needed anything like a formal discussion about sex, birth control, or sexually transmitted diseases. Their whole lives, subjects that are generally discussed only behind closed doors at their friends' houses were normal dinner table fodder in our home. And since I'd been a midwife, they overheard many of my phone conversations with clients.

Colin, my fourteen-year-old son, had invited a friend over for dinner and to spend the night. We were awaiting his arrival when Colin approached me while I was preparing spaghetti.

"Mom?"

"Yes?"

"Um…well…"

"What?"

"If you get a call from some patient during dinner tonight, could you go upstairs to talk to her?"

"I guess so. But why?"

"It's just that… I don't know, maybe I'm wrong, but I don't think that Neil is ready to hear you asking some woman whether her bag of water has broken, what her vaginal discharge smells like, or when was the last time she had sex."

"Ah."

"Yeah, you know, stuff like that. His mom sells real estate. I mean, she's not a midwife. Neil's kind of quiet, maybe a little shy. He probably should get out more, but whatever. Anyway, I just don't think he's ready to overhear a conversation about vaginal discharge. It might traumatize him for life."

"Right. I'll definitely go upstairs to use the phone tonight."

Big and Little

When she was still six weeks from her due date, Nicole developed a low-grade fever; then her bag of water broke and her temperature shot to a dangerous level. As she was clearly a very sick lady, my backup doctor immediately performed a Cesarean on her. The baby weighed less than five pounds and wasn't released from the hospital for more than a month.

Breastfeeding was difficult from the beginning. The baby was tiny. She had a hard time latching on and a weak suck. With so little sucking stimulation, Nicole wasn't making much milk, and she became very discouraged.

About the time Nicole's baby was sent home, I attended the home birth of another woman's second baby. The mom, Hannah, pushed out a bruiser of a boy, a chunky kid who weighed more than ten pounds. This burly baby had the sucking power of an industrial Shop Vac, and Hannah had so much milk that she began donating to the Mother's Milk Bank.

Then I had a "storm of brains," as my older son once called his bright ideas: Why not introduce these women to each other so they could perhaps swap babies for mutual benefit? They lived only a couple of miles apart, so I did it.

For several weeks, they met daily to nurse each other's babies.

Nicole's breasts reacted to the power-suckling of the big baby boy, and her milk supply quickly increased.

Hannah donated her surplus milk to Nicole until Nicole's supply matched her daughter's needs.

Nicole's baby learned how to suckle properly at Hannah's breast by getting an immediate letdown of abundant milk with minimal effort.

Gradually, Hannah's breasts stopped producing quite so much milk, because Nicole's baby didn't stimulate the milk nearly as aggressively as her own son did.

Since that initial bonding experience, the two women have

remained friends to the present day. Both babies thrived.

Much as it would have made a fairy tale ending to the story, the babies did not, however, grow up to marry one another.

But two other babies I helped into the world *did* end up marrying each other…

Three Births and a Wedding

It was a busy morning in April of 1983.

I had returned home at 2:00 am but slept only half an hour before leaving to be with Josie, a mom having her second baby. She was well along in labor upon my arrival, but then she stalled. I examined her, and she was nearly fully dilated.

But – and it was a big But – her bag of water was intact and the baby was floating high in her pelvis. To break the amniotic sac might possibly precipitate an umbilical cord prolapse, one of the true emergencies in obstetrics. Most definitely *not* something that's "fun" to deal with even in a hospital, let alone at home. I'd been there twice before, and I was in no mood for a replay.

So we were kind of stuck, wanting for Josie to resume active labor, but not wanting to break her bag to force the issue. Any minute it would break on its own. Or not. It was a dilemma.

Then, Laura, a first-timer called, and she was also in labor. She didn't sound particularly active yet; she was just giving me a heads up. But her bag of water had broken, and she said there was "some meconium in it."

What to do, what to do?

I looked around the scene at Josie's. Bonnie, a longtime family friend of Josie and John, and Sandi were both with me. I figured they had it covered, and at least for the moment, Josie was in a sort of suspended state: very close to giving birth, but also very much *not* in active labor. So I held my breath, crossed my fingers, and zipped back to Laura's house in central Berkeley.

I turned onto Doug and Laura's street just past Berkeley Bowl, the iconic former bowling alley turned into a grocery store. It's one of the several "typically Berkeley" places I take out-of-state visitors for a Show and Tell. I remember my first awestruck visit there many decades earlier...standing in the doorway and staring at fifteen varieties of apples, twelve kinds of mushrooms, an olive deli bar at which sampling of the twenty different offerings was encouraged, and about fifteen kinds of organic salad greens in open bins. I remember thinking, How on earth do people *choose?* Berkeley Bowl is sort of a destination, a museum. So much more than "a grocery store."

Half a block down a side street, I parked and walked toward Doug and Laura's. They lived in a small cottage at the rear of a pretty stone courtyard that they shared with a few other families. Not exactly a "commune," just an urban communal space in The Village Berkeley.

I knocked, and Doug opened the door. Morning light streamed through the window, and a black cat slept on the tidy bed. Laura looked serene and radiant, dressed only in a black T-shirt and a pair of underpants. She had a hand towel stuffed inside the panties.

Indeed, there was meconium in the fluid, but it was watery, and the baby's heartbeat was strong. I stayed through several contractions – still mild – and the baby's heartbeat remained steady, so I assured them I'd be back in about an hour or so, as soon as Josie's baby was born, and I left.

No problem.

Back at Josie's house, I stayed...I stayed and I stayed and I stayed...and she just wouldn't get into productive labor. But I was reluctant to leave, because my money was still on Josie giving birth as soon as I turned my back. And once her baby was born, there would be plenty of time for me to return to Laura's, not more than ten minutes away. I would leave Bonnie behind to stay with Josie and her newborn for a couple of hours, and I'd take Sandi with me to Laura's.

That was my plan. It was a good one. A reasonable one.

Except that Josie just would *not* get a move on, and a couple more hours dragged by.

Then things changed.

Doug called and said, "Laura's in the shower, and she's making barnyard sounds. And she just told me her body's pushing, all by itself. Also, a lot more water is coming out, and now the fluid is really dark brown, and it's thick."

Doug was usually a pretty cool customer, but it sounded as though his *sang-froid* had deserted him. Finding himself at home with a wife bellowing in the shower, a baby about to be born, a lot of meconium in the amniotic fluid...and no midwife on the premises was more than he'd bargained for.

I said, "I'm on my way."

He shouted, "I'll unlock the door. Hurry," and he hung up.

Laura was climbing out of the shower as I arrived, bloody show and thick meconium running down her legs. She had that *the-baby-is-coming-right-now* look on her face and didn't make it all the way to the bed before another powerful contraction hit her...and the head was visible.

In spite of the intensity of her labor, Laura was very, very calm. Her composed and serene face was surrounded by clouds of dark, curly hair. She was in a trance.

Doug was not. He was on high alert, tense and wired, wanting to do something. Anything.

As Laura sank to the floor, I barely had a chance to grab a basic birth pack from my supplies before the baby's head landed in my hands, eyes open but very pale. And I could see the umbilical cord wrapped tightly more than once around her neck.

Moments later, the rest of the baby somersaulted out, and there she stayed, in my hands but snug against her mother's perineum. The cord, tangled around the baby, wasn't long enough for me to move her at all.

And she didn't look great. Limp. Breathless. Pale, pale, pale...and utterly gift-wrapped in the umbilical cord.

The cord twined twice around her neck, across one shoulder, and all the way around the body of the baby, who must have been doing yoga inside the uterus to get so tangled up. Usually when the cord is wrapped every which way from Sunday like this one, it's a very long cord...but Laura's baby's cord was average length, so it was pulled taut, and I had no room to maneuver.

Eventually, I rolled and flipped the baby girl this way and that, loosening enough of the cord to unwrap her all the way, and then I went to work. With anxious fingertips, I felt her chest for the heartbeat, and it was present but quite slow. I began breathing for the baby, and while she didn't cry or make any attempt to breathe on her own, her heart rate rose almost immediately to a normal rate.

Laura lay still. She held her head up with both hands so she could watch, and a dreamy look of complete certainty that All Will Be Well spread over her countenance.

Doug, without the benefit of Laura's hormonal trance, breathed deeply, asked desperately what he could do to help, and looked very frightened – with good reason, in my opinion.

I kept breathing into the baby's nose and mouth, and between breaths asked Doug to open my oxygen tank and turn it on. He did, and I put the tubing in the corner of my mouth so the air I was giving the baby had more oxygen in it that my own exhalations could provide. The cord was pulsing, so the placenta was still playing its part in the resuscitative effort, too.

At about the three or four minute mark, Sarah – for that's what they named her – squeaked, then gave her first cry, and finally began breathing on her own. I kept the oxygen blowing on her face for several more minutes as she continued to rapidly improve.

After we'd all calmed down and gotten Laura and the now pink Baby Sarah settled between clean sheets, I sat back, took a deep breath, and began to do a little charting. There wasn't much to write, as I hadn't even been present for the labor itself, but I carefully calculated the Apgar score.

Babies are routinely scored at one minute of age and again at five minutes. The Apgar score is not done immediately after the birth, primarily because it's not relevant: a lot happens physiologically and chemically as babies transition from living underwater to living in the air, and they deserve at least a minute to allow those changes to occur before somebody slaps them with a score card.

But even making allowances for these factors, I didn't feel justified giving Sarah a score higher than two when she was a minute old. She had a good heartbeat at that point.

And not much else. One minute into her life, she was still limp, still pale, still not breathing, and still not responding to stimuli.

But I gave her eight points at five minutes, subtracting a point each for tone and reflexes, and a score of eight is just fine. Certainly by ten minutes of age, she was a perfect ten on the chart.

But it had been unsettling for all of us, and we needed a bit of time to catch our breath. I called Sandi to let her know what had happened, and she said Josie seemed to be picking up some momentum. I asked her to come stay with Laura and do the newborn routines, and when she arrived, I headed back to Josie's. [4]

* * *

---

[4] Josie's highly unusual and ultimately hilarious birth is related in the chapter titled "Push Me Pull You" in my previous book, Midwife: A Calling.

Three years after Sarah's dramatic and somewhat alarming entry into the world, Laura again gave birth at home.

Margaret Love, a personal friend of Laura and Doug's, was my assistant and apprentice for that birth. The couple had moved from the small ground-floor one-bedroom cottage where Sarah had been born to a second-floor flat on the same piece of property...and when we arrived together, Margaret stared up the steps in amazement.

"I used to live here," she said. "That flat is where my son was born," and for the zillionth time the thought occurred to me that Berkeley is more like a hamlet than a city. The interconnectedness of the residents seems to acknowledge no boundaries. It's not Six Degrees of Separation at all; it's more like three. Maybe two.

It just felt right that Margaret should catch Laura and Doug's baby. On the floor again, Laura appeared relaxed and smiling. Labor progressed quickly – no surprise there! – so I mostly just sat back and watched. On Laura's third push, the baby slid into the hands of a joyfully laughing Margaret. Then Laura and Doug began laughing, and so did I. No stress. No rush. No sweat. Just happiness.

This time it was a boy, Paul, and best of all, he screamed upon arrival and scored nine at one minute and a perfect ten at five minutes.

* * *

Six months prior to Paul's birth, in March of 1986, I had caught Brenda's second baby, and *caught* is really the right word.

When Avi, Brenda's husband, called me, he said, "She seems to be going really, really fast this time. You've got a bit of a drive ahead of you, and honestly, I'm not sure you're going to make it."

I put in a quick call to Margaret to meet me there, and I started off. I made it, but it was quite a feat of fancy driving. Curtsying briefly at stop signs and sliding through a few orange traffic lights, I sped north. I turned left into the woods of Kensington, then left again down a narrow drive among towering firs and redwoods, passed under what looked like a medieval town gate, and pulled to a stop beside the little Hobbit cottage where they lived. The house looked like it belonged in a movie, an artificial creation of a Sixteenth Century rural village, missing only a few gnomes and fairies peeking from behind the ferns.

Margaret pulled in right behind me. Hurrying up the crooked stone steps, I tried the door, found it open, and together we hustled to the

167

bedroom…

…and found Brenda brushing her teeth.

I stopped, put down my gear, and said, "Sooo, what's up?"

Brenda didn't answer, just kept brushing her teeth.

"She's been brushing her teeth ever since I called you," said Avi. "She only started having contractions a couple of hours ago, but… wow."

Then I noticed Brenda's knees were crossed, there was a wet spot on the floor between her legs, and she was staring at the wall with intense concentration.

"You ready?" I asked her. "Feel pushy?"

She nodded, spat out a mouthful of toothpaste, rinsed her mouth, hobbled over to the bed, lay down…and gave birth to Gabrielle. Margaret made the catch, actually, because she was closer and quicker than I was.

When a labor and birth happen like that, there's really little need for a midwife at all. As such times, I feel virtually superfluous. One of the skills of a midwife is knowing when to sit on your hands and when to act. Most of the time, with the addition of a few whispered words of encouragement, a suggestion of a change of position, and a bit of guidance during the birth, there's a lot of sitting on hands happening.

And this was one of those times. As I drove home a bit later, I pondered what a small role I had actually played.

But that changed about twenty-five years later.

* * *

Brenda got in touch with me and told me her daughter, Gabrielle, was engaged to Paul.

To say I was delighted is putting it mildly. And very surprised.

"How did this happen?" I asked her.

Avi and Doug, the two dads, had coached the junior soccer teams that their kids played on, and they became friends. They'd both played the game themselves as youngsters, so, realizing how much they missed it, they started a casual adult game on Sunday mornings. Soon a Wednesday evening game was added, and the events became a unique and special tradition between their shared communities.

After the Sunday games, a bunch of the guys always went to a café for breakfast, and in time, over coffee and home fries, Avi and Doug discovered several unique similarities: they had both taken childbirth classes from me, their oldest kids had been born a day apart (although Ilann, Brenda's first baby, had been born in the birth center at Alta Bates), and they'd both had home births with Margaret Love and me.

Twenty years passed. Brenda and Laura knew each other socially from events related to their husbands' love of soccer. Talking together one afternoon, they realized both of their children were about to graduate from college and would be returning to the Bay Area.

And they talked some more and discovered that neither of their kids was involved in a serious relationship at the time. They looked at each other. They smiled. And a plan was hatched.

Brenda told Gabrielle they were all invited to a barbecue at Doug and Laura's house, but Gabrielle was suspicious. She remembered Paul, but they hadn't really spent any time together since they were kids.

"You're not planning to try to fix me up with someone, are you?"

"No, no. Of course not. There'll be lots of people there."

So Gabrielle, still wary and reluctant, agreed to put in an appearance.

Of course, when the evening arrived, only six people were present: Gabrielle, Paul, and both sets of parents…and shortly after dinner, the parents melted into the fog rolling in off the Bay, leaving the young couple alone in the yard.

They had talked long into the darkening evening…and now I was being asked to marry them.

"Oh, yes," I said, "I'd be delighted. Honored," but then I paused. "Um, you're all Jewish, right? But me? I don't know from Jewish."

"Yeah, but they don't want a Jewish wedding. They just want it to be meaningful. We've all been trying to think who to choose to perform the ceremony, and it was actually Gabrielle who thought of asking you, as you were the link through which they connected in the first place."

"Done!"

So, on the twenty-third of June 2012, my husband and I drove to the wedding venue at the Headlands Center for the Arts in Marin County. Milling around among the guests while waiting for the service to start – and weddings always start late, right? – I discovered that, in addition to the bride and groom, also present were three other "babies"

I'd caught. One was the wedding planner's assistant, and another was the daughter of one of the guests. Also, Laura pulled me over and introduced me to Sarah, the one who had scored two on the Apgar score when she was a minute old.

A tall, slim, lovely young woman put out her hand, and I shook it as I looked with delight into her beautiful eyes. Laura then pulled me aside and said, "She just got her MBA, so I think she's fine, don't you?"

I have to admit to being relieved.

Not much later, I found myself standing before about a hundred guests with Paul at my side, and together we watched Brenda and Avi lead a nervous Gabrielle down the aisle toward us.

As part of the ceremony, I shared with the guests the serendipitous events that had led up to the wedding day, the Berkeley-as-a-village impression that was symbolized by this union, and the parental plotting that had brought the two young people together. And my own pleasure at once again being asked to share an important event in the life of these two families.

As the bride and groom turned to face their friends and family, I concluded the service with the following:

"From this day forward,
you shall travel the world as a couple.
You shall be together
even in the silent memory of the ages.
But let there also be spaces
in your togetherness.
So let the winds of joy forever dance with you,
between you, and around you.

By the power vested in me by the state of California
it is with great honor and joy that I now present to you all
Gabrielle and Paul."

Two years later, in November 2014, Gabrielle gave birth to her first child, a daughter named Clementine, at the home she shares with Paul in San Francisco.

And thus the circle was completed.

All White

Renée always wore white. It didn't appear to be a religious or a spiritual thing with her. It just seemed to be her preferred color. Okay, there was the occasional cream shirt or very pale beige slacks, but really: white. I figured it sure must make outfit coordination simple when she opened her closet every morning.

Tommy, her husband, came to several of the prenatal visits with her, and while he wore khaki pants, I never saw him in anything other than a white business shirt or T-shirt.

But when I did the prenatal home visit at around the thirty-fifth week of her pregnancy, I could hardly see them in their own living room. Talk about camouflage: they disappeared into the background because absolutely the whole house was white.

White walls, white wall-to-wall carpeting, white furniture...even the teacup she handed me on a white plate was white.

At least the cookie on the plate was dark brown, a delicious gingersnap.

But I thought, Wow, I almost need sunglasses around here.

Tommy and Renée were in the business of house-flipping; they bought houses in so-so condition (but in good neighborhoods with good schools) for below market value, spent money bringing them up to code, painted everything white, added a minimal amount of modern white furniture, and put the house back on the market as quickly as possible. They lived in each house while working on the next one, keeping two sets of furniture in use at all times. Renée said it took about six months for each house, and so far they had more than doubled their money on five houses.

I was impressed. By the time I met them, they'd amassed a tidy little fortune, especially for a couple who weren't even thirty and hadn't yet had their first child.

I admired some modern art on the wall above the white leather couch. There were three shadow boxes in soft gray wooden frames, and in each was a collection of twigs, each bound with either silver wire, white ribbon, or tan raffia. They really were lovely: calm, serene, natural. I suppose an interior designer might have called them "minimalist organic."

Tommy smiled and said he'd gone looking for stuff to hang on the walls for the first house they flipped, and he found boxes of twigs similar to these at a designer showcase for $500 each.

"I figured, shoot," he said. "Twigs and white ribbon? I ought to be able to make those myself." He went to Jo-Ann's and Michael's craft stores where he bought the shadow boxes and Plexiglas, plus wire, raffia, and ribbon. "Then I walked down the street and picked up twigs from the lawns and sidewalks between here and the corner. I spray painted the frames, then got to work with the twigs and stuff."

He said his first couple of attempts were clumsy, but by the third or fourth try he'd gotten the hang of it. "They ended up costing me about ten bucks apiece, and I figured that was a lot better than the $1500 it would have cost me at the art studio. So I've been making all our wall art ever since. Just from stuff I find up in Tilden Park, in the Sierras, or, like these, right here on our street."

I figured if or when the California housing bubble burst, he could make a living with twigs and white ribbon and probably do just fine.

As I nibbled my gingersnap, I mentioned the havoc a toddler might potentially wreak on the all-white theme, but Renée said, "Everything's washable, and I think white is the easiest color to deal with because you can just bleach everything."

Okay, then.

A week past her due date, Tommy called me and simply said, "She won't come out of the bathroom. I think it's time." I could hear Renée squeaking, trilling, and sort of clucking in the background, so I left immediately.

When I got to their home out in Walnut Creek, a suburb on the other side of the hills to the east of Oakland and Berkeley, I found Renée still in the bathroom. All white, of course. Her long blond hair hung in a loose ponytail down her back. She wore one of Tommy's old white T-shirts and stood barefoot on the white shag throw rug.

A roll of toilet paper sat on the white tile counter.

She looked at me, gave me a quick smile, then rose to her tiptoes as another contraction began. She reeled off about six feet of toilet paper, wadded it into a little ball, and began scrubbing obsessively at a nonexistent spot on the counter. The wastebasket overflowed with perhaps fifty of these crumbled balls of tissue that she'd already "used." Of course, as the counter was already spotless, the tissues in the wastebasket were entirely clean.

As she scrubbed, she began making noises that sounded like a songbird, a chicken, and a cat trying to harmonize – or maybe settle an argument. Either way, it didn't sound as though they were having much success.

I called Margaret. Even without examining Renée, I could tell she was entering the final stages of a pretty quick labor, considering the size of her belly. Also, I had unwisely made an assumption that was quickly proving to be untrue.

What with the white house, the white furniture, and the white clothing, I suspected there might be a little OCD going on, perhaps just some tiny issues with control, possibly germ phobia…I had anticipated Renée might have trouble "letting go," getting down and funky, engaging in the primal and fascinating free-wheeling process we call Childbirth.

Clearly, I was wrong. She was busy, focused, sweating, intense… very much at one with the process. She was on the birthing train, and she had found her rhythm: wiping the counter and chirping.

I laid out my supplies on one end of the long and now cleaner-than-ever countertop. I could see the bedroom just around the corner, and it had been prepared for the birth. But I had the feeling Renée had already grown some serious roots in the bathroom, and I was pretty sure nothing short of a national emergency would budge her from her chosen venue.

Tommy stood in the doorway, and beside him was a Costco-sized bag filled with rolls of toilet paper. He said, "She's already gone through four rolls, all we had in the bathroom cupboard, so I just went out to the garage and brought the whole bag inside."

By the time Margaret arrived, Renée's hair had come loose and was hanging over her face. As I was wiping it back and re-tying it into a ponytail, she pushed my hand away, kicked the white rug out the door, and squatted on the white tile floor. Margaret yanked the plastic off the bed and brought a pile of towels into the bathroom while I opened my small package of sterile supplies.

Suddenly Renée put her hand between her legs, backed up and

173

eased herself onto the toilet. The moment she took her hand away, the bag of water broke and splashed into the toilet.

"Tidy," said Margaret. "Very tidy."

We laid a few of the towels and some Chux on the floor while Tommy just watched, mouth agape, from the doorway. Renée clung to the toilet with one hand and the edge of the bathtub with the other, and within fifteen minutes she pushed a huge baby into my hands.

Renée sat down on the towels, leaned against the bathtub, and took her son into her arms.

"Tommy, would you get the baby blankets from the oven, please?" I asked, and he zipped off, reappearing in seconds with a foil-wrapped package of receiving blankets. All white, of course. We finished drying off the baby, put a cotton cap – white, what else? – on his bald head, and wrapped him snugly in a couple of oven-warm blankets.

Renée cooed to him, Tommy entered and climbed into the dry bathtub to peer over his wife's shoulder at his husky newborn.

Then Renée got a funny look on her face, said, "Uh-oh," and scooted the baby into Margaret's arms. She slid up and onto the toilet again, and in seconds the placenta plopped into the toilet water.

"Yep, very tidy indeed," said Margaret.

The kid looked to be a good ten pounder, and Renée didn't even have any skid marks. A few minutes after the placenta came out, after we'd fished it out of the toilet, and after we'd clamped and cut the cord, Renée asked Tommy to turn on the shower. With the hand-held attachment, she hosed herself off, then put on a pair of adult Depends, a clean white T-shirt, and walked into the bedroom where she settled herself between clean white sheets and began to nurse her baby.

It took Tommy, Margaret, and me about thirty seconds to erase all traces of a birth having occurred in the bathroom.

We examined the baby, weighed him – officially ten pounds, nine ounces – and measured him, took Renée's blood pressure and kept an eye on her minimal bleeding, did some charting, and after eating at least half a dozen more gingersnaps, we were on our way home about three hours after I'd arrived.

"One of the tidiest births I've ever seen," said Margaret as she got into her car.

"And the whitest," I said, as I got into mine.

A Good Man is Hard to Find

My husband, Rog, can do nearly everything I do. That would probably include catching babies in a real pinch, although it's never been tested.

He can cook, change diapers like a pro, take care of car maintenance or at least get the cars to a shop to have routine stuff done (I call it 'well-baby care,' like lube and oil, rotate the tires, stuff like that), wash dishes, do laundry…

He can't breastfeed, of course. I remember coming home one afternoon from work, years before I was a midwife, to find our firstborn vigorously sucking on Rog's thumb knuckle, absolutely the only thing this baby would accept other than a human nipple. No pacifiers, no rubber nipples, no pinkie…

It was rough sometimes, I'm sure, and that day Rog handed the baby off to me, sighed, and said, "I'd give anything to have breasts right now. Seriously. My kingdom for just a single tit would be great."

He's not so good at folding laundry, actually, and he doesn't load the dishwasher properly, i.e. the way I think it should be loaded, of course. But really, he's tremendously versatile. Years ago, someone asked Sandi, "What does Roger do?" and without missing a beat, she replied, "Whatever's necessary."

And it's true. I knew if I left in the middle of the night, he might or might not be aware I'd even gotten out of bed, but if a situation with our children arose and he found my side of the bed empty, he would uncomplainingly handle whatever needed doing.

The phone rang one night when Skylar, was three. Our third and final *au pair* had returned to Scandinavia two months earlier, so we were on our own.

A ringing phone and my quiet conversations with either hospital nurses, laboring moms, or anxious dads had long since ceased to waken my husband, so he slept on as I answered the phone.

A baby was coming. I slid out of bed, dressed quietly, tiptoed downstairs, put my shoes on, grabbed my gear, and left the house.

The baby was birthed with ease, at least from my point of view, and I was home shortly after sunrise. I slid carefully into bed, not wanting to disturb my husband, but before I'd fallen asleep, Skylar entered our bedroom.

One look at him, and I knew both he and my husband had had a rough night. The poor kid was gray, and translucent blue circles rimmed his eyes. He looked haggard, and his hair was damp, perhaps from fever. A sicker, more miserable-looking little boy I'd rarely seen.

Without a word, my husband rolled into a sitting position...and I saw he was naked. This is a man who never, ever sleeps naked, a man who loves his pajamas and bathrobe and slippers with a zeal bordering on passion. Besides, it was March, and it was cold. Before I could question this naked man about his state of undress, our gray-faced son spoke for both of us.

"Daddy, why you no got no jammies on?"

Rog's shoulders slumped a bit before he answered. He sighed deeply, then said, "Well, Skylar, it's like this. You threw up on one pair of my jammies, and you shat on the other pair. And I've only got two pair of jammies."

I tried not to, I really did...but I howled with laughter.

Rog, who surely knew I'd left during the night, as he'd had to deal with a sick toddler all by himself, whipped around and stared at me. "When did you get home?"

"Only five minutes ago. I'm probably in better shape than you are, though, so stay in bed and I'll handle things for the next few hours."

It's a Boy...

Monica's husband, Abel, had a genetic condition that he didn't want to pass on to future generations, so they agreed they would use donor sperm, and conceive their baby by artificial insemination. They purchased the semen from a local sperm bank, brought it into the office, and I did the insemination.

They really wanted a girl badly, so, to increase their odds of that happening, they came into my office three days before Monica expected to ovulate.

Here's the deal:

Boy-sperm move faster but die off more quickly.

Girl-sperm move more slowly but live longer.

So if couples want a boy, they schedule the insemination as close to ovulation as possible, hoping a speedy boy-sperm will outpace the slower girl-sperm and be the first to reach the ovum ambling along somewhere up in the Fallopian tube.

If they want a baby girl, the insemination should be performed a few days before ovulation is anticipated, on the theory that most of the boy-sperm will have died off by the time the ovum is released, and lots of longer-living girl-sperm will still be hanging around, just lying in wait.

The insemination procedure was fun. Joyful, even. They were both there, holding hands, and I was thinking, Wow, maybe I'm about to impregnate this woman...

First I moistened my fingertips with some of the semen and rubbed it onto Monica's cervix.

Next, using a large syringe, I sucked up the semen and attached a skinny catheter, a little wider than a cocktail straw, to the tip of it. I pushed the tip about ¼ inch into Monica's cervical opening and injected some of the fluid directly into her cervical canal.

Monica had brought her diaphragm along, at my request, so I spread more of the semen around the rim and slipped it into place. Then I fed the end of the catheter over the lip of the diaphragm and injected the rest of the sample right into the rubber cup itself.

Abel put four pillows under his wife's hips to elevate them and keep her cervix in contact with the pool of semen in the diaphragm – and she stayed like that for half an hour.

I went into another exam room to continue caring for my pregnant clients, but I could hear Monica and Abel giggling behind the closed door. I smiled, because maybe there actually *was* a baby being conceived in there.

Yup. It worked. She missed her next menstrual period, and the pregnancy test came back positive.

Everything progressed normally, and Monica remained convinced she was carrying a daughter. All the old wives tales agreed with her prediction, the Ouija board said it was a girl, and people on the street – total strangers – frequently smiled at her and said, "I'll bet you're having a girl."

When Bonnie and I arrived at her house in the Oakland hills, Monica was chugging along in pretty good labor. Her sister and her mother were also there, along with several close friends. Video cameras were pretty new at the time, but Abel had purchased one and was excited to be using it to tape the birth of their first child. This was well before the era of digital video recorders, and his contraption was large and unwieldy.

I was concerned that his focus through the camera lens would mean he would forfeit his own participation in the experience, but I needn't have worried. As Monica advanced into late labor, he handed the bulky camera to one of their friends, showed him which buttons to press, and warned, "Careful with how much you film now, cuz we're eventually going to run out of time. I want to be sure there's enough time left on the tape to capture the actual birth."

His friend nodded, checked the time remaining…and as the next couple of hours passed, I could see he was paying attention, turning the camera off for long periods to save room for the birth itself, as well as the joyful moments right afterwards.

Monica pushed like a champ, working in harmony with her body. Abel was attentive, totally in tune with her wishes and needs. He whispered encouragement to her, wiped her sweaty brow with a cold washcloth, supported her when she tried squatting for a while, and even peeled off his clothes to get into the shower with her.

At last the baby's head began to show, but it was one of those slow ones, like two steps forward and two steps back, making excruciatingly slow progress, nearly invisible progress, with each contraction.

Back and forth, back and forth the baby rocked. As the heartbeat was dropping quite low during contractions, I suspected we might be dealing with either a short umbilical cord or a cord artificially shortened by being tangled around the baby.

We worked in different positions, and eventually having Monica lie on her right side with her top knee sharply flexed onto her belly seemed to steady the baby's heartbeat to a happier rate. This position also proved to produce quicker descent of the head.

Hank, the guy holding the video camera began to look anxious, constantly checking how much time was left. He probably hadn't expected such a lengthy and problematic pushing stage.

"Got another tape?" he asked Abel. "This one's getting pretty close to the end."

"No, that's the last one. How much time is left?"

"About eight minutes."

"Oh, jeez. Just shut it off until the baby's actually coming out."

I told Hank I'd cue him when I figured only a couple of contractions remained. And I did...so the camera didn't begin rolling again until the baby's head truly crowned.

With the next contraction, the head came all the way out...and I could see several loops of cord around the neck.

Bonnie turned on the oxygen tank while I tried to loosen up at least one of the loops to provide a little slack. But it was no use. The cord was tight, tight, tight. The baby's face was dark purple, and the cord wouldn't be budged.

The camera rolled on as, with the next contraction, the child's head stayed right next to Monica's perineum while the rest of the body somersaulted out – completely wrapped in the cord, including loops between the legs, over the shoulder, and around the body.

"It's a boy," shouted someone near the head of the bed...

...and Hank said, "Whoops, tape just ran out."

"That's okay," said Abel. "At least you got the birth."

But I was far too busy to worry about the video recorder. I had more important things on my mind. I untangled the baby from the many loops of what turned out to be a very long umbilical cord, and then Bonnie and I went to work trying to get the child jump-started, for this was a very listless and very pale little kid. Deep purple head and pale gray body. Not a good combination.

Then Monica began to bleed. I left Bonnie to deal with the baby, and I turned my attention to delivering the placenta. As I was coaxing the afterbirth to cooperate, I heard Monica say, "It's a boy?" and several people answered in the affirmative.

"Really?" she said. "I was so sure it was a girl…"

"It's fine, honey," said Abel. "We'll have a girl next time," but I could tell both of them were a little disappointed.

Finally the baby gave a lusty cry and began to turn the right color, and then the placenta slid out, albeit reluctantly. But Monica had what we call a lazy uterus. It didn't want to stay contracted on its own, so I started an IV and put Pitocin in the bag. Someone took it from me and hung it from the light fixture on the wall at the side of the bed.

We had all been very busy for quite a while, but after about half an hour, at last we could start to relax. Monica cuddled her swaddled baby, and Abel curled up beside her to admire his son. Monica's mother disappeared and returned with a bottle of champagne and a pan of brownies, and we had ourselves a little party.

Finally I asked Monica if she was ready for us to weigh the baby and do a quick physical exam, and she handed the squirmy little bundle over to me. She sat up to watch as I unwrapped him and prepared to measure his head circumference, but I paused…

…and I turned to the group of people still crowded around the bed and asked, "Didn't someone say it was a boy?"

"Yeah, I did," said a guy next to Jesse.

"Well, um…it's a girl."

"*What?*" shouted Abel.

"*What?*" shouted Monica.

"*What?*" shouted everyone.

I turned the baby around to face her parents so they could see for themselves. It was definitely a baby girl.

Everyone began laughing except Monica, who began crying. "A girl, oh my God, it's really a *girl*. Oh, Abel, it's a girl, a girl. We have a *daughter!*"

Billy, the guy who had prematurely – and incorrectly – announced the baby's sex was mortified and said, "I don't understand. I swear I saw a penis as soon as he, I mean she, was born…"

"The kid had the cord between her legs, and I'm sure that's what you saw. You're not the first person to be confused," I reassured him.

We partied on with even more enthusiasm after this surprise discovery, but then Hank said, "Uh, guys, I just thought of something. The tape ran out right after Billy shouted 'It's a boy.' How are you going to explain this video to your daughter when she's older? She'll probably think she was adopted or switched out for another baby or something. She'll think she was a changeling."

"Oh, wow…" murmured Abel.

Everyone looked puzzled, mildly concerned, worried. Could this actually be a problem for them and their daughter in the future?

Then I had an idea. "Look," I said. "What about this? Run the tape back, and then end it or cut it or erase it, whatever you have to do, but make the tape end right before the sex is announced. Would that work?"

Abel thought for a few seconds, smiled, and said, "Yeah…yeah, I think I can do that. That should work just fine."

As Bonnie and I left with the gaggle of friends about an hour later, Abel and Monica, and her mother and sister were still exclaiming, "Wow, a girl, can you believe it, really, it's a girl, a girl, a girl…"

A Piece of Poop

Poop happens.

Whatever is in the lower bowel during late labor will most certainly be expelled as the mother pushes her baby out.

It's natural, it's normal, it's common…and everyone in the profession of catching babies has learned to deal with it discreetly and efficiently.

But back when I was training as a student nurse in the early Sixties, a Triple H enema (high, hot, and helluva lot) was routine for women admitted in labor. This was the era in which a lot of effort was put into trying to make childbirth "sterile." During those days, a simple vaginal exam (which, if the bag of water is still intact, is now done with a clean – but not sterile glove) was a really big deal: the mother was scrubbed, put in stirrups, and draped as if she were about to have major abdominal surgery. The doctor put on a mask, scrubbed his hands (they were all men then) – exactly as if he were going to perform surgery – then donned a sterile gown and sterile gloves.

Really.

All in an effort to preserve the "sterility of birth."

Never happened. Never gonna happen. *Clean* is about the best you can aim for, but sterile?

Uh-uh.

But not for lack of trying. In addition to the enema, women also routinely had every scrap of pubic hair removed. In reality, the nicks that occasionally resulted from the obligatory shave made women more liable to infection, which was the exact opposite result of the original intention.

And let's not even talk about the itching that occurred as the hair grew back. And the scratching. Yeah…

I hope no hospitals still follow these embarrassing, infantilizing, useless, and potentially harmful practices, but even into the mid-Seventies, there were a few doctors at Alta Bates who still insisted on the shave and enema.

From vast experience, allow me to say that a piece of poop is a lot easier to deal with at birth than the residual results of an enema that has become trapped behind the baby's descending head and that then blows out explosively at the moment of birth.

Give me a little piece of firm or semi-solid poop any day.

Dierdre's first birth dragged on for an incredible three days. It was one of those nasty ones that starts out with about thirty-six hours of prodromal labor, the wheel-spinning nonsense that produces minimal progress and maximal exhaustion. Contractions too weak and too far apart to produce dilation, but too close and too uncomfortable to allow the mother to sleep.

By the time real labor finally kicks in, sometimes both mother and baby are too fatigued to handle the situation with much success.

These are the cases in which a dose of morphine to stop the contractions and permit the mother to sleep is often the most humane approach. Another option is an epidural and Pitocin; once the mum is pain free, it's hoped she can sleep, then waken in late labor to participate actively in her child's birth.

But I was still strictly a home birth midwife without hospital privileges when Dierdre's first baby looked like she was going to take a month of Sundays to come Earthside. Morphine or an epidural with Pitocin weren't options for my clients unless they transferred to the hospital.

So Dierdre soldiered on with the loving help of a rotating group of friends and family, and finally...finally...her daughter was born at home.

Damned if her second – and her third – labors weren't almost as long. It just wasn't fair.

So when labor began with her fourth child, we were all geared up for another record-breaking ordeal.

However, just two hours after his first call letting me know maybe labor was starting, Teddy, Dierdre's husband, called me and said I'd better hurry up, hurry up, hurry up, "the baby is coming *right now*, right this minute."

Well.

Hurry I did, but I still missed it.

While the small bedroom looked as if a ferocious battle had been waged and won, the atmosphere was actually pretty peaceful by the time I arrived. I kicked aside towels and sheets strewn all over the floor, slipped in a puddle of amniotic fluid, then reached the bed where Dierdre, looking like she'd just watched a truck suddenly crash through the wall of her bedroom, lay sprawled with her squalling baby in her arms.

"I felt like I had to push," she said, "but I *knew* it couldn't be the baby. Not *this* fast. So I stood up to go to the bathroom. And the baby just came flying out. Flying *out!* I mean, I was standing up, and I don't know…if Teddy hadn't been right there, I guess she'd have hit the floor."

Teddy was prowling around the room, peering into corners and muttering something that sounded to me like *poop…poop…*

He interrupted his pacing and turned to his wife. "Nah, you'd have put your hand down there, I'm sure you would have," he said. "No way you'd have let her hit the…" but his voice trailed off. He looked distracted as he lifted a towel, shook it out, and tossed it into a corner.

"What are you looking for, Teddy?" I asked him.

"Poop."

"What?"

"Poop. There's a piece of poop around here somewhere."

"What do you mean?"

"Well, there's a little piece of poop around here somewhere, I swear. Just a little piece. Dierdre's poop, not the baby's…yeah, a piece of poop came out as the baby was born. Dierdre was standing up, and I just caught the baby and the poop at the same time. But I tossed the poop away somewhere. I didn't want it. But I don't remember where I threw it. And now I can't find it."

"Don't sweat it, Teddy," I said. "I'm sure it's just among the sheets. I'll help you clean the room up after we get Dierdre and the baby settled."

"But it's here somewhere. Just a little piece of poop."

"Relax."

"But…it's poop," and he resumed his hunt.

"Teddy," said Dierdre. "Chill out."

I checked Dierdre and the baby, delivered the placenta and cut the cord. Then Dierdre took a shower while Teddy and I finally tackled the business of tidying up. The whole time we worked, creating order out of chaos, Teddy kept muttering, "… just a little piece of poop, it's around here somewhere, poop, poop…"

Finally I was ready to leave. Teddy helped me schlep my supplies outside, and he loaded them into my car for me. Then I went back inside to arrange for a home visit the next day and to say good-bye to Dierdre. I gave her a hug, picked my purse off the floor where I'd tossed it upon my arrival and swung it over my shoulder.

"Uh!" I heard Teddy give a little triumphant shout. He was staring at me.

"What?" I asked, mystified.

"Aha! I *told* you there was a piece of poop around here," he shouted, and he pointed to my purse.

Stuck to the bottom of my green purse was, yes, the missing piece of poop.

Just a little piece.

But Teddy was so pleased with himself.

Me? Not so much.

The F Bomb

Lila's first birth had been textbook perfect. Steady progress, no snags, no pauses, no complications. From the time of her first inkling that "something might be happening," as she said when she first called me, until she showed signs of advanced labor took only about seven hours. As if they were following a script, the contractions predictably became stronger and closer together as the time quickly passed. She walked around her small house in Oakland's flatlands for most of that time, and soon a thick rope of bloody mucus appeared on her thigh. She wiped it off, tossed away the tissue, and continued pacing.

Then she grunted at the height of a contraction and looked at me, startled.

"It's the beginning of pushing," I reassured her. "Let me examine you to be sure you're fully dilated." Everything was so utterly normal that I didn't really expect to find a thick anterior lip of cervix ahead of the baby, or even a thin rim…but I didn't want her to add voluntary effort to her pushing until she was completely dilated.

She stood in front of me as I checked her. No cervix was palpable, so she was good to go, and she instinctively headed for the toilet.

And that's where her bag of water broke. So convenient, so tidy. A quick glance told me the fluid was clear, so I checked the baby's heartbeat and just sat with my back against the bathtub and watched her carry on.

Then, without saying anything, she stood up, grabbed a bath towel off the rack, held it between her legs, and waddled to the bedroom.

"It's fine if you stay on the toilet," I assured her, because she looked so comfortable there.

"No," Lila said as she arranged pillows and Chux pads on her bed, "when I tell this kid about its birth, I don't want to have to say we fished him out of the toilet."

Her second stage, the pushing part, was also steady and efficient. Forty minutes later, she was staring into a mirror Margaret held up for her so she could watch the descent of her baby's head. It was as if she'd stepped onto a conveyor belt at the onset of labor and was then steadily carried along like a mechanical toy. Only instead of a Jack-in-a-Box, there would be a real live baby at the end of this assembly line.

About fifteen minutes more of spontaneous pushing were all Lila needed before reaching down between her legs, grabbing her son under his armpits, and pulling him up to her chest.

Lovely. Just lovely.

She named him Wolf, after her grandfather.

Because she was breastfeeding her son on demand, her menstrual periods didn't return – which is entirely normal. Like many other women, she assumed she wouldn't have to worry about birth control as long as she wasn't menstruating.

It's true…sort of…only not really.

The trick is that you ovulate two weeks before you menstruate. A menstrual period tells you that you didn't get pregnant two weeks ago. But the *lack* of a menstrual period can mean one of two very different things: either you're still not fertile – or you ovulated two weeks ago and are now pregnant again.

That's what happened to Lila. She didn't realize she was pregnant with another baby until her nipples began to ache when Wolf nursed – and they hadn't bothered her at all since the first few days of nursing him when he was a newborn. Then she lost her taste for coffee and good French cheese. And then she vomited one morning.

So, although they weren't planning another baby for maybe another year or two, it was really okay, as she'd been planning on weaning Wolfie in a few more months anyway, so she could get pregnant again.

She and her husband discussed the option of having Wolf around during the birth, and, because of how very smoothly her first birth had played out, I thought it'd be fine. But ultimately Lila made the decision to have her mom take Wolf off to a park – or, if it was the middle of the night, just stick around in case he woke up and then take him off to her own house. Lila didn't want to feel inhibited by his presence, and she didn't want to frighten or confuse him. She just wanted freedom to do her own thing.

She called me when she felt she was beginning to move into the active phase of labor. In reality, she was already there and had called me a bit too late, not to put too fine a point on it. When I arrived, she was in the shower, but I heard her making those typical very late labor noises as soon as I walked through the front door.

I went into the steamy bathroom, pulled the shower curtain aside, and noticed copious bloody mucus on her thighs. I watched as she clung to her husband, and then she bent into a crouch with the next contraction. I didn't bother checking her, just went into the bedroom and started setting out my supplies.

Gramma was patiently trying to slip the arms of a very reluctant toddler into a jacket and persuade him to leave the house with her.

He wasn't buying it.

He wanted a different jacket, he wanted some juice, he wanted a banana, and he wanted his green truck. Gramma couldn't find the "right" jacket, she wasn't sure where the juice boxes were, and she could find only his red truck. She did find a banana, but that wasn't enough to appease Wolf. Not nearly enough.

He dawdled, he whined, he stalled, and then he collapsed on the floor with the banana clutched in his hand...and Gramma was desperate.

Lila came out of the bathroom wrapped in a towel. She stood at the entry to the living room with her legs crossed at the knees and her toes curled. On her face was a look of steely determination, and her mouth was contorted into a rictus of a fake smile.

She stared at Wolf, and in a strained voice, she promised him "a trip to the Little Farm in Tilden Park" the very next day if he would "Just. Go. With. Gramma."

Wolf turned his eyes up to his mother and didn't move.

"*Now*, Wolf. *Right this minute.*"

He got the message. Gramma, Wolf (in the "wrong" jacket), and the now-squished banana finally headed out the door.

As soon as the door shut behind them, Lila screamed, "*FUCK*" at the top of her lungs. Then she took three giant leaps and launched herself toward the bed – where the baby was entirely born with the next contraction. I grabbed the infant from midair, right before she would have landed at the edge of the bed. I bobbled her once, then got a good grip on her.

I had to assume the baby was crowning while Lila had been having that "conversation" with her son.

While I was still rearranging the speedy airborne baby in my hands and untangling her from the umbilical cord, Jeff leaned over, opened the window facing the front yard, and hollered, "Hey, Gramma, come on back."

Looking understandably confused at what she thought was a sudden change of plans, Gramma returned, leading Wolf by the hand, and the two of them stared at Lila holding the squalling baby girl.

"You have a little sister, Wolfie," said Lila.

Gramma was completely nonplussed; she hadn't even had time to unlock the car door. "When? What? But..."

Lila, looking immensely relieved, said, "Yeah, it was crazy fast. She was born with the very next contraction, right after you left."

"Mercy," said Gramma, looking discombobulated.

I was a little discombobulated, too. I don't think I'd done a mid-air catch before. Lila hadn't even completely landed on the bed, much less settled herself properly, before the baby flew out.

Lila's husband, however, looked like his wife gave birth explosively every day and twice on Tuesdays. One very cool dude. He went outside, fired up the barbecue, and began to cook ribs for all of us.

But Wolf was even more pragmatic than his dad. He showed the barest smidge of interest in the new baby. He was much more concerned about washing squashed banana off his hand, finding that missing green truck, and nailing down the promise his mother had made just five minutes earlier.

True to her word, Lila and Jeff loaded Gramma, Wolf, and their newborn daughter into the car the very next day, and they drove to Tilden Park at the top of the Berkeley Hills - and Wolfie got to pet some bouncy baby goats.

The Coagulation Shuffle

Paula seemed like a perfectly ordinary woman, a mother of four young children. Nothing in her demeanor or conversation led me to believe she subscribed to any of Berkeley's many off-the-grid belief systems. She held a graduate degree in history, and her husband was an executive in an investment company in San Francisco. They lived in a large two-story house in the Berkeley hills, right on the border with Kensington, a small upscale neighborhood in which nearly every home had a panoramic view overlooking San Francisco Bay. Picture postcard images of Berkeley's waterfront, the glistening bay dotted with sailboats, ferries, and freighters, San Francisco herself, three bridges, and the Pacific Ocean beyond the Golden Gate Bridge drew one's gaze toward the many west-facing windows in Paula's house.

During the middle of her pregnancy, Paula's hemoglobin level was 11.5, so I prescribed iron supplements for her, along with some dietary suggestions. The level wasn't dangerous, just a bit on the low side of normal. As babies draw from the mother's iron stores as pregnancy progresses, I wanted to be sure Paula had enough hemoglobin left for her own wellbeing. Without supplementation, we would expect to see her level decline into the truly anemic range of 10 or lower.

Some people believe a woman who's anemic in late pregnancy is more likely to hemorrhage, but that's not true. What *is* true, however, is that an anemic woman who hemorrhages will get into trouble more quickly, as her iron stores are already depleted. To be certain the hemoglobin levels improved or at least held their own, we retested moms around six to eight weeks before term.

But Paula had somehow slipped through the cracks, and it wasn't until two weeks later that I realized I had missed it. I ordered the blood test immediately, asking her to do it that very day, but I was confident, as I assumed she was taking the iron supplements, that she'd be in the safe range.

When the results came back the following day, I was shocked. Her hemoglobin had actually dropped to 9.8, putting her below the level at which I would do a home birth. My limit was 11.0. Less than that, and I would deliver the mom only in the hospital.

I called, told her she was anemic, and I asked her what kind of iron pills she was taking.

"Well..."

Oh, dear lord, what now? I thought. "What? Have you been taking them, or haven't you?"

"Well..." she repeated. "I see an alternative nutritionist, and she said I didn't really need to *swallow* the pills in order for them to work. They can cause constipation. She said I just needed to absorb their *essence*."

"Their *essence*. Okay, how did you absorb their essence?"

"Three times a day, I picked up the bottle of iron pills from the kitchen windowsill and held it in my fist. I closed my eyes and meditated on their *essence* flowing into me."

"Oh."

"Is that bad?"

"It didn't work. I can't deliver your baby at home unless you actually start *swallowing* those pills three times a day, every single day. Maybe four times on Sundays. I want you to take them on an empty stomach, before meals, but take them with a glass of orange juice to aid absorption. You need to increase your iron count significantly before you go into labor, or else we'll be doing this birth in the hospital."

I also talked to her again about adding iron-rich foods at every meal. I knew I'd made an impression on her, and I assumed she would comply. I just hoped she didn't go into labor a couple of weeks early.

Two weeks later, her hemoglobin had risen to 10.8, still low but heading in the right direction. A week later, it was 11.1.

Okay, I'd have loved it if she'd been 12.0 or 13.0 – but at least it was rising steadily now that she was actually swallowing the pills and not just absorbing their freaking *essence*. To be on the safe side, however, I had her see Joe Weick, my backup doctor, mostly to get his blessing to go ahead and deliver her at home.

Joe said if she carried the pregnancy another week, continued with the supplements, and followed a good diet, her level would probably rise to at least 11.5, and he was fine with that, so we went ahead with plans for a home birth.

Labor began eight days later. Confident her hemoglobin was heading in the right direction, I had no qualms as I headed up into the hills to her house.

Paula wanted a water birth. At the time, the terrific rental tubs that have now become so commonplace didn't exist, so she planned to use the bathtub. I wasn't yet a big fan of water births, mostly because I'd done only a few of them, but I agreed – on one condition: when the baby emerged, I really didn't want to engage in a contest to see how long we could keep her underwater.

I'd seen some videos of babies bobbing and floating underwater for what felt like forever before being lifted into the air. It's true that babies instinctively hold their breath when their faces are in contact with water. It's also true that babies, in theory, don't need to breathe room air as long as the placenta is attached and fully functioning.

When the placenta begins to detach from the uterine wall, there are some classical but often subtle signs, and there's usually a little fresh vaginal bleeding.

Usually. But not always.

So if the baby is being kept below the water for some reason such as a desire to capture a video of her "swimming" happily for a few minutes (which in my mind always seem to stretch to infinity), it's possible the separation of the placenta might be overlooked…in which case, the baby will probably gasp for air.

And inhale water instead.

I just didn't want to go there.

But Paula was fine with my conditions and agreed that as the baby was born, she would reach down and guide her from the water and onto her own chest in one smooth, fluid, and continuous movement.

There was another slight snag in the plan. I'm incorrigibly right-handed. It's never a problem if the mother is squatting, standing, or on all fours. But if a woman is reclining, I will move furniture, dogs, kids, and other people out of the way in order to place myself on her right side.

Paula's bathtub, the only tub in the house, had the faucets and spout on the left end of the tub, and I needed only one glance at it to realize she would be lying with her head at the other end – which would position me on her left side.

My brain and hands won't coordinate with each other that way, so

I knew I'd be taking my shoes and socks off, rolling up my pants, and straddling her in the tub at the time of birth.

And that's what we did.

Really, however, as things transpired, I was superfluous. It all went so smoothly that I mostly just watched as a beautiful underwater birth unfolded naturally.

Margaret Love was assisting me that evening, and she helped me shift Paula and her newborn daughter out of the tub after the placenta was expelled. We settled Paula in her bed where she began breastfeeding her daughter, and we started tidying up and putting our supplies away – very few of which we'd actually used.

The baby checked out perfectly as we weighed and measured her, did a physical exam, and dressed her in a diaper, a shirt and a soft cotton cap. Then we swaddled her in warm receiving blankets.

Paula wanted something to eat. We offered to get it for her, but she wanted to do it herself. An hour or more had passed since the birth, her uterus was firm, and she wasn't bleeding much at all, so no problem. Up out of bed she rose, pulled on a pretty robe, and walked down the stairs to the kitchen. She fixed scrambled eggs, tea, and English muffins for all of us. I carried it back upstairs for her, and we had a tea party with some celebratory champagne at the end.

Two hours had passed, Margaret and I loaded our supplies into all their boxes and bags and were in the process of saying goodbye when Paula got a strange look on her face.

"I think I just peed myself," she said.

I pulled back the covers…and she was hemorrhaging. Already a puddle of blood spread from her waist to well below her knees, and it began dripping off the side of the bed.

I grabbed for her uterus and began massaging vigorously, but it was already hard as a rock, just as it should be. The uterus contracts after the birth to minimize bleeding from the site where the placenta was previously attached…and Paula's uterus was contracting perfectly. She hadn't torn during the birth, so I couldn't imagine where the blood was coming from. Margaret took over uterine massage while I opened my supply boxes again, the ones we'd been about to carry out to my car.

I opened the oxygen tank, turned it on, and put the mask on Paula's face. I then examined her with a speculum to see if I could spot a cervical or vaginal wall tear or a big hematoma. It was difficult to halt her bleeding long enough for me to see very well, but everything I saw appeared normal.

"Come here, Andy," I said to Paula's husband. "Hold her feet and legs up in the air," and he did. Pale-faced, scared, and speechless, he kept it together pretty well under the circumstances.

I called 911, then started an IV, knowing we would be going to the hospital and also knowing she would need a transfusion. This was just way, way, way too much blood for her to lose.

Blood is thick and won't flow through a skinny needle, so I used a big bore needle and put three ampoules of Pitocin into the IV bag. Pitocin is used to contract a sluggish uterus, and while Paula's uterus was far from sluggish, I knew it couldn't hurt and, frankly, I didn't know what else to do, under the circumstances.

As soon as the IV was flowing well, I phoned Dr. Elizabeth Clark, who was on call for Joe Weick that night. The answering service reached her quickly, and I told her we'd be arriving by ambulance, bringing in a woman with a postpartum hemorrhage.

Still Paula bled.

Margaret was vigorously massaging the already firm uterus, holding it between both her hands and rubbing and squeezing – to no effect. Pitocin and IV fluids poured into Paula – to no effect. I took her blood pressure once, and it was 80/50, where previously it had been 120/70. She was going into shock, looking paler by the minute.

The paramedics arrived – and they were a home birth midwife's worst nightmare. They discounted me, dismissed me, ignored me, and scorned me.

Then one of the guys looked at the IV and asked, "What's in the bag?"

"Three amps of Pit," I said and then watched in horror as he removed the IV. Not just switched out the bag, but the whole IV apparatus, needle and all.

"What are you doing?" I shouted. "She's going into shock, and that was a perfectly good IV with a big bore needle."

"We can't take your word for what's in the IV bag. We have to start it ourselves."

"That's crazy," I yelled, trying without success to control my rage and fear. "You could just have hung a new bag if you really needed to, but you sure as hell didn't need to remove the needle."

But it was pointless. By then my IV was toast. They swabbed her pale, freckled arm with alcohol and tried to get a new IV started, but her veins had begun to collapse. They finally got a skinny little needle into her hand, useless for giving blood.

They took their sweet time taking Paula's blood pressure and temperature and counting her pulse. They asked pointless questions about her medical and obstetrical history. *No*, I wanted to scream, *she doesn't have diabetes or heart disease!*

I was frightened. I was also incensed, and becoming more so by the moment.

Eventually I shouted, "Just stop! Do all that while we're en route to the hospital. She's hemorrhaging, and the doctor is already there and waiting for us."

"We're following protocols. Stand aside. Her, too," the guy in charge said, referring to Margaret, who was still elevating and massaging the uterus. At least they let Andy continue to hold Paula's legs up.

Margaret stood back, but the EMTs didn't take her place. I was pretty sure Paula wasn't bleeding from the placental site in the uterus because her uterus could *not* have been firmer. But it's routine to massage the uterus of a hemorrhaging woman…and these guys didn't seem to think it was important at all.

I began to wonder exactly what protocols they *were* following… and if they even comprehended the extreme gravity of the situation.

As their blood pressure reading also revealed impending shock, they searched among their supplies while I fumed at the valuable and life-saving time that was passing. Already they'd been at the house for fifteen minutes, and the hospital was at least a twenty-minute ride away. Eventually they pulled some inflatable shock socks from their supplies and, pushing Andy aside, hauled them onto Paula's legs way up past her knees. Then they inflated them. The purpose is to impede blood flow to a patient's legs, increasing blood supply to the more vital organs in the brain, chest, and abdomen.

Finally, finally, they opened the gurney, lifted Paula, and placed her on it, leaving behind a bed that was now totally saturated in her blood, not to mention another quart or so on the floor. I looked at the scene for a moment, and dots swam before my eyes.

I had never before seen so much blood at a birth in all of my more than two decades of experience.

As the crew entered the hallway, they realized the stairway turned twice, and the angles were too tight to permit the gurney to go down intact. So they broke it down and converted it to a chair, raising Paula's head and lowering her legs.

She immediately lost consciousness.

I was horrified, but perhaps for her it was a blessing: she did not regain consciousness until hours later and remembered nothing beyond that point.

More than twenty critical minutes had passed before they at last slid Paula into the ambulance. Her husband climbed in beside her, and I followed.

A beefy arm blocked my way. "No. Only her husband," and he started to close the door.

"Massage her uterus and lift up her feet and put some Pitocin into that bag." I hollered, and the door slammed.

Margaret and I shared a horrified glance before we got into our cars and sped after the ambulance. Paula's sister, who had been present throughout the birth and all that followed, stayed behind with the baby and the older children. My last glimpse toward the house was of her standing in the open doorway, both hands to her mouth.

We burst through the doors of the OB department at Alta Bates at the same time as the men steering Paula's gurney.

"What took you so long?" Dr. Clark growled. I took a deep breath, rolled my eyes, and jerked my head toward the ambulance attendants. The doctor took a good look at Paula, gray and unconscious, then pulled me aside as Paula was wheeled into the OR. "I thought you were bringing me a hemorrhaging woman, not a dying one," she said.

Wow.

It was as bad as I feared. As bad as it could possibly get.

Andy took a seat in the corridor, and Margaret sat beside him. He sank his head into his hands; Margaret put her arm around his shoulder and began whispering to him.

The anesthesiologist miraculously managed to start two good IV's, drawing several tubes of blood for lab work at the same time, and someone called the blood bank for as much O-neg blood as was available. People with O-negative blood types are called "universal donors;" although rare antibody reactions have occurred, in theory, almost anyone may receive O-neg blood without precipitating a transfusion reaction.

Tom Churchman, another obstetrician, had delivered his own patient by Cesarean just half an hour before our dramatic arrival. He, too, rapidly assessed the gravity of the situation. As he was already scrubbed for surgery, he donned a fresh sterile gown and gloves and then stood against the wall of the OR with his hands clasped above his waist.

He just stood there. He didn't say anything. He didn't do anything. I looked at him and raised my eyebrows in a silent question. He moved a little closer to me, careful not to contaminate his sterility by touching me, and he said quietly, "Hard to say which way this will go. I thought I'd stick around in case Elizabeth needs to operate. Or if she just wants someone to bounce ideas off of. Or if *you* want to unload. I mean, you must have had a helluva night."

I nodded and managed a weak smile.

What a kindness. By now it was 2:00 am. No light at the end of the tunnel. Dr. Churchman was giving up a night's sleep while expecting no remuneration, even hoping he wouldn't be needed at all...but he was willing just to hang around for moral support, offering an extra pair of hands, or, if necessary, a shoulder to lean or to cry on.

I prayed I wouldn't need to cry on his shoulder.

Elizabeth examined Paula thoroughly and found exactly the mystery that had confounded me: there was no obvious reason for her bleeding. No uterine atony. No lacerations in her cervix, vagina, or perineum. No hematoma on the vaginal wall.

Yet she steadily bled. Two bags of blood and other blood products and one of saline (into the IV started by the ambulance guy) were pouring into Paula. Dr. Conway, another obstetrician who happened to be there that fateful night, began making repeated trips to other hospitals in the East Bay, returning with her arms loaded with blood and blood products.

Still Paula bled with a steady and audible drip, drip, drip.

And it totally and irrevocably sank in: Paula was dying. Five children, including a newborn, would be raised without their mother. I, a home birth midwife, was about to experience the unheard of: a maternal death. How that would impact me and the other midwives, not to mention Paula's family…it didn't bear thinking about.

And I realized I was going to faint.

I backed up unsteadily, intending to lean against the wall and slide to the floor, but I bumped against a stack of risers [5] and sat down heavily. I lowered my head between my knees.

Tom came over, said, "You okay?" and I shook my head. He left, then returned with a cup of strong sweet tea and an ice-cold washcloth. He handed me the tea, wiped my face with the washcloth, then draped it across the back of my neck. I held the tea and drank it. The sugar, the caffeine, and the jolt of scalding fluid brought back my vision and stability.

As soon as he saw I was improving, he stripped off his now contaminated gown and gloves, donned fresh sterile ones – and resumed his quiet watching and waiting.

I heard the anesthesiologist say, "Pink ink," and we all knew what he meant. Paula's blood was so diluted that her body was living mostly on only IV fluid with a little blood mixed in. The blood that she was hemorrhaging was pale pink.

And she wasn't clotting. DIC, disseminating intravascular coagulation, had set in. DIC is a life-threatening situation in which a widespread clotting cascade is activated in the small peripheral blood vessels, depleting clotting factors elsewhere in the body. If unchecked, it leads to diminution of blood to the vital organs and eventually to multiple organ failure and death.

The anesthesiologist looked at me and jerked his head. Glad to be asked to do something, anything at all, I went over to him.

"Call the ICU and ask Marilyn to come down. I'm sure she's on, because I saw her up there earlier tonight. Tell her to bring her gum because I need a subclavian line put in, and she's way better at it than I am."

"Gum?"

"Yeah. Just do it. She'll know what I mean."

A subclavian line is a large catheter that's inserted into a really big vein just below the collarbone. It's used for rapid drug and fluid infusion and monitoring of central venous pressure, among other

---

[5] Risers are stackable lifts designed to elevate shorter nurses to the height of taller physicians during surgery.

things.

I called the ICU, and about five minutes later a short, no-nonsense nurse bustled into the OR with her arms full of supplies, and she quickly assessed the situation. She pulled a big pack of chewing gum from her pocket, handed it to the anesthesiologist, and then set to work, first wiping orange Betadine over a wide area beside Paula's neck.

I couldn't see most of what she was doing, but periodically she said, "Gum," and the anesthesiologist unwrapped another piece and put it in her mouth.

I was mystified.

In about ten minutes, she was finished. The vital line was securely in place and functioning. By then, Marilyn had five sticks of chewing gum in her mouth. She bundled up all the leftover debris from the procedure, tossed it into the trash, and was on her way back up to the ICU.

"Wow," I breathed. "She's fast. And good. But, um, what's with the gum?"

"Don't know for sure," the anesthesiologist said, shaking his head. "She's really, really terrific at placing these lines, but she can't do it without fresh gum being constantly fed to her. She always carries plenty. We've all just gotten used to it. Something about meditation, distraction, concentration. I don't know. I just know, for her, it works."

Another hour passed. We'd been in the OR for four hours. Paula was unconscious, but only lightly so, because she responded to pain by flinching and moaning. She'd been given only 25mg of intravenous Demerol, and although everyone would have liked her to be anesthetized for this ordeal, we knew more of any narcotic, anesthetic, or sedative would probably kill her.

Elizabeth, Dr. Clark, took a step back and looked at Tom. He moved closer, and I heard her say, "I might have to do a hysterectomy, although I have no idea where she's bleeding from or why. But if I do a hyster, she probably won't survive the surgery. Yet if I *don't* operate, she'll *definitely* die. What do you think?"

"Tough call. She's right on the edge now. I think you ought to try surgery, but honestly? I'm not sure."

"I'm going to operate," she said.

She walked toward the door to obtain consent for surgery from

Paula's husband, but she stopped and turned back. Almost as if she were talking to herself, she muttered, "Wait, let me…I just…maybe there's one more thing…"

She took a long thin spinal needle and drew up a large dose of prostaglandin, a drug used to control postpartum hemorrhage. She swiped an alcohol swab right above Paula's pubic bone, then plunged the needle in deeply and injected the medication. It reminded me of an iconic scene from the movie *Pulp Fiction*, although that long needle had gone into the heart of Uma Thurman, whereas this one went into Paula's lower belly.

Still.

I turned away. I've never liked to watch long needles enter body cavities. I can handle virtually anything medical or surgical, but I don't like watching spinals or epidurals given. I never liked to watch an amniocentesis to collect a sample of the amniotic fluid. I don't like watching fluid drained from chest cavities or from the heads of hydrocephalic babies. I've observed and/or assisted with all of them multiple times, but it always makes my toes curl.

And I definitely didn't like seeing that very long needle go deep into Paula's belly.

I was still looking at the floor when I noticed Tom Churchman's feet begin a weird little dance. Two steps forward, one to the side, two steps back. Shuffle, shuffle, kick. Repeat.

"What the hell are you doing?" I whispered.

"It's called The Coagulation Shuffle. Shhh. I think it's working. Can you hear it?"

I listened, I listened hard.

And then I heard it.

Plop.

The drip-drip-drip of blood seeping from Paula's body had turned to a soft plop…and then another one. Plop…plop…plop.

She was clotting.

Finally.

The bleeding stopped entirely within a few minutes. But it still took an hour before she was stable enough to leave the OR and be moved to the ICU, where Marilyn took over her care.

I accompanied Paula up in the elevator along with Dr. Clark. "What exactly did you do?" I asked.

201

"It was just a stab in the dark. Literally," and she gave a little bark of laughter at the dark humor of her comment. "I realized the only place we really couldn't check for bleeding was the lower uterine segment, that no-man's land between the cervix and the upper part of the uterus. So I just injected prostin right into it. If it hadn't worked, I'd have operated, and I'm pretty sure she'd have died. But she was dying anyway, so it was worth a shot. I still can't believe it worked so quickly."

Paula remained in critical condition in the ICU for a week before moving to the postpartum floor for another three days of convalescence. Then she went home. She still had her uterus. Her husband still had his wife.

And her five children still had their mother.

Second Thoughts

After Paula's near-disastrous birth experience, my body recovered from the stress and the endlessness of that long night, but my mind, my heart and soul, most definitely did not.

I – and everyone else involved – had spent five hours in the operating room, waiting to see if Paula would live or die. Two obstetricians, an anesthesiologist, two nurses, and I had kept a fearful vigil. Paula's husband stayed with Margaret in the hallway for all those long and anxious hours. Periodically he stared through the small window into the room where his unconscious and ashen wife, surrounded by a lake of blood, lay flat on the table with four IV lines running into her.

The third obstetrician, Dr. Conway, had made multiple trips between Alta Bates and all of the other hospitals in the East Bay, greatly depleting their blood banks' supplies. Indeed, as I was later informed, she *did* completely eliminate the stock of Type O-neg blood that night, and she made heavy inroads into type specific O-pos blood, plus packed cells, serum, coagulation factors…

She took anything that might be useful, anything that was handed to her. She put these bags of precious and potentially life-saving blood products into a Styrofoam cooler, set it beside her in the front seat of her car, and hurried back to Alta Bates. Time after time after time.

The memories of those hours flooded relentlessly back to me, and I wakened several times each night with a racing pulse. So when Cynthia called me two days later and told me her labor had started, my heart thudded and faltered. It was her third baby, and she planned a hospital birth. There was no reason to expect a problem – yet a part of me wondered if I could really continue doing this job.

But midwifery is far more than a job. To most of us who find ourselves catching babies, it's really not a job at all.

It's a calling.

I had long ago answered that call – and never doubted that I was doing exactly that which I was meant to do.

But now, I doubted.

I didn't doubt that I was meant to do it, nor did I doubt that I *could* do it.

I wasn't sure that I *should.*

Paula's postpartum hemorrhage had been so bizarre, so atypical, so inexplicable, that intellectually I knew my reaction wasn't realistic. Yet the blood loss had been so torrential that, just remembering the scene, dots swam before my eyes and I grew dizzy all over again.

Two full hours after the birth, Margaret and I could so easily have already been on our way home when the bleeding started. And although the behavior of the ambulance crew was actionable, in my opinion, and had contributed to Paula's dire condition upon arrival at the hospital, I hated to think what might have happened had we not still been at her house when the hemorrhaging began.

For the first time in my career, I was relieved that I wouldn't be called upon to attend a home birth. Cynthia was headed to the hospital, and in the hospital, doctors, nurses, anesthesiologists, an operating room, and the blood bank were within seconds or minutes away from each labor room. And the intensive care nursery was just down the hall, should it be needed.

I arrived at the hospital about fifteen minutes after Cynthia checked in. She had waited at home, laboring with her husband and sister, until contractions were strong and regular at three-minute intervals, so she was already seven centimeters dilated upon admission. A perfectly smooth and normal birth of a healthy baby girl followed within the hour.

Nothing was needed except calmness and confidence. The obstetricians weren't needed, nor the OR, and not the intensive care nursery. Most definitely the blood bank wasn't needed. The hospital itself was superfluous, except for it being the place where Cynthia felt most comfortable giving birth.

Yet I was glad it was over, and I was glad she'd chosen the hospital instead of her own home. Looking at Cynthia sitting up in bed, nursing her chunky nine-pound daughter with all the usual shiny chrome equipment surrounding her, I wondered if I would regain enough confidence to attend home births ever again.

As I was heading to the dressing room to change out of my scrubs, I met Dr. Conway in the back corridor.

She smiled, reached out, and touched my arm. "How are you doing?"

This was not a woman who had ever been particularly supportive of me. She wasn't unsupportive or antagonistic. Just neutral. We had rarely had a conversation of more than a couple of sentences since I'd started attending births in the hospital.

I was surprised at her obvious concern for my well-being, and I was grateful. I *wasn't* doing well, and I knew it.

Dr. Clark and I had had a long conversation when we met in the ICU where Paula was still in critical but stable condition, but it was mostly a technical exchange, not really deep on an emotional level.

Yet here was this doctor who had stayed up all night with no thought of anything other than the fragile life of an ashen woman – a woman she had never met – lying limp on the operating table. She had worked for hours to help prevent the death of a patient who had been delivered at home by the first midwife to whom the hospital had granted privileges.

As she looked into my eyes and waited for my reply, I knew she was sincere, and I knew she wouldn't walk away from an honest answer.

"No, I'm really not okay. I'm pretty freaked out, actually," I finally said. "There's a part of me that thinks maybe I should go back to trade school to become an electrician or a plumber. Some line of work as far away from midwifery as possible. I'm not sure I can do this any more."

"Well, that would be a mistake."

"You think so? That woman almost died."

"Yes, indeed she did. That's as close as I've ever seen someone come to dying, someone who didn't go on and actually die, I mean. But…"

"Don't say it wasn't my fault," I interrupted, "because, intellectually, I know it wasn't anything I missed or did wrong. It's just…"

Then it was her turn to interrupt. "No, I wasn't going to say that. Of course everyone has heard about it, and everyone is talking, but no one is blaming you. It's surprising, actually, because I know there wasn't universal support for giving you hospital privileges. I think everyone knows it could have happened to any of us. Yes, it's unfortunate that time was wasted in the transport from home to hospital. But that was a very, very, very rare situation, and I still don't know how it occurred to Elizabeth to do what she did – which most definitely saved that woman's life."

"I know, I know, but…"

"No. No Buts. You can't live your life trying to avoid all the extremely rare situations that Fate could potentially throw at you. If you give in to it, fear like that will paralyze you. You could live four lifetimes and never again see something like this. Rare complications are *rare*, trust me."

She pulled me into an empty labor room and we sat on a small couch as she continued. "But it's something else, isn't it? Realistically, you know this won't happen again. What's wrong?"

I hesitated to say it. Most obstetricians don't "approve" of home births, and a few have gone to the insulting extreme of saying, "home birth is a form of child abuse," so I was cautious. I really didn't know where she stood with regard to home birth.

But, in for a penny, in for a pound. What did I have to lose?

"I'm wondering how I can get the courage to continue doing home births. For the first time, when I came in to catch a baby a couple of hours ago, I was relieved she had chosen the hospital. I was incredibly relieved that I didn't have to face doing another home birth. I'm honestly not sure if I could have done it. I might have invented some reason for her to transfer to the hospital – and if I'm feeling like that, then I should stop doing home births."

There. I'd said it. I'd stated the unimaginable.

"I thought you might be thinking along those lines. I saw your face in the OR, and you were almost as pale as that woman lying there on the table. But I'm going to say again what I said in the first place. That would be a mistake."

"Why?"

"Why? For all the obvious reasons. Some women will insist on having their babies at home. That's always been the case and always will be. They're often the ones who fear doctors and hospitals – with all the rigid protocols – more than they fear the relatively small risk of a home birth, and their fears aren't necessarily misplaced."

I'd seldom heard a doctor speak so frankly on the subject, and I'm sure she saw my eyebrows rise.

"Don't look so surprised. I'm aware that some of our routines are superfluous, and that sometimes, just by following these routines blindly, we create those very situations that lead to more and more interventions. It's like dominos falling, and I understand why there are women who will choose an out-of-hospital birth rather than put themselves in our path. I'm not particularly in favor of home birth, but I'm a realist. If that's what they're going to do, then I want them to be as safe as possible."

I was really warming to this usually aloof doctor, so I said, "For sure. Many of my clients fear the results of unnecessary intervention far more than they fear not being here should a complication arise."

"I know. And while I don't entirely agree, I do understand their reasoning."

"You know, it's so unusual for me to have to bring someone from home into the hospital for an emergency. A transfer is almost always initiated because of prolonged labor and exhaustion."

"Yes, but that's pretty much exclusively a first-timer's problem, isn't it?"

"Sure, although, as we have both just witnessed, the profound complications – postpartum hemorrhage and prolapse of the umbilical cord – don't follow that rule."

"True," she said, and by this time I was beginning to feel as though I was talking to a colleague, not a doctor I scarcely knew.

"In those cases, the very least obstetricians can do," she continued, "is be supportive of the midwives who are willing to attend home births. *We're* not going to do it, us obstetricians, so there *must* be midwives available who have the experience and skill to manage the complications that sometimes – rarely, but sometimes – will occur."

I nodded, but half my brain was thinking, Yeah, but why me? Let some of the new ones take over, and I'll just hide out here in the hospital.

"From my perspective, you're obligated to pass on your knowledge, your judgment and your skills, to the rafts of midwives who are sure to follow you. The gates are open. You've paved the way. Carry on, my dear, so that others may be as well received as you have been."

"Oh, jeez, thanks for that, but…" and I sighed.

"No, I'm serious. And it's probably like what they say about falling off a horse. The best thing you can do is to climb right back on again." She nodded her head and gave my arm a couple of pats. Then she stood up, said, "You'll be alright," and she walked away.

I sat there for maybe half an hour…not thinking about anything in particular, just allowing what she'd said to trickle through the filters and barriers I'd erected.

When I finally rose and went to change my clothes, I realized that, with the conversation I'd just had, I was already in the process of talking myself back up onto the horse again.

Three days later, I was called to attend a home birth. Margaret arrived within minutes of me, and together we climbed the steps to the front door.

I rang the doorbell. Before the door opened, we looked at each other and took a big breath. A really big breath.

When the door opened, we smiled and stepped inside.

No No No

Louisa's pregnancy had been very stressful, filled with loss and fear and sadness. When she was just three months pregnant, her mother suddenly died of a ruptured aneurysm, and two months later Gordon, her husband, was diagnosed with a serious melanoma. He had completed chemotherapy just a few weeks earlier. Then, when she was seven months pregnant, her cat had to be put down after being mauled by a raccoon. And her sister had surgery for breast cancer.

She said, "Enough. Enough sadness. Enough loss and pain and fear. If this baby is a girl – and I think it is – we'll name her Olivia. It means Life."

Early in the pregnancy, Gordon, a contractor, embarked upon a modest home remodel: a master bedroom and bath were to be added, plus a new living room, which would involve repositioning of the front door. All this would be completed in plenty of time for the baby's arrival.

As happens with many remodels, especially when the owner of the house is a contractor with big dreams, one thing led to another. It seemed that the bigger Louisa's belly grew, the bigger the house plans grew. But dealing with the effects of chemotherapy had slowed Gordon down. And, while pregnancies have a finite ending, construction projects often do not.

Louisa voiced her concerns about the status of her house during one of her prenatal visits. She said, "Now he's gutted nearly the whole house. I'm serious. The kitchen's gone, and the master bedroom is just roughed out with chalk. No roof. And he's torn down the stairs.

"We're staying in a small downstairs bedroom, and he's working like a dog, but I don't think it's going to be in very good shape anytime soon."

I drove by a few weeks later to take a look for myself – and she was right. It had been raining, and one dismantled exterior wall lay in the mud. Heavy plastic sheeting stapled to four-by-fours served as a temporary "wall," and I could see plastic flapping at the rear of the house, too. I assumed it was the "roof" of the proposed master bedroom suite.

It looked far from promising, but Gordon assured Louisa and me that "enough will be finished in time for the birth."

I wondered what his definition of "enough" might be, suspecting the heavy rains we were experiencing had thrown a serious monkey wrench into his plans.

Another few months passed and it was time for me to make a prenatal home visit, a chance for me to see the interior of this big project and to find out exactly what I would soon be dealing with.

I parked and walked along narrow planks laid atop gloppy mud; I could hear it sucking and releasing with each step I took. At one point, mud crept over the edges and stained the sides of my shoes.

Holding a handsaw, Gordon opened the door for me, but he disappeared and went back to doing manly things when Louisa appeared. I looked around, then looked at her. She gave me a rueful glance, shrugged her shoulders, and said, "Um, yeah. Let me show you around."

And really, the house was in a shambles. The walls of the existing bedroom were down to the studs, and they seemed to be living out of a row of cardboard boxes filled with their clothing. The temporary stairway had treads but no risers. And no railing. It looked kind of like a ladder laid at a slant.

The kitchen was completely gone. A sheet of plywood on two sawhorses held a microwave, an electric kettle, and a stack of plastic plates and utensils.

As I looked around, it was obvious that nothing had really been completed…and the baby was due in less than a month.

I couldn't imagine anyone choosing to give birth in such a setting. Really, it looked like a refugee encampment, and not a very sturdy one.

Gordon reappeared, saw me staring at what looked to me like barely controlled chaos, looked sheepish, and hastened to reassure me. "There's still a month before the due date, and I've got my energy back. And maybe the kid will be late."

Having been involved in some large remodeling projects myself, I knew the best laid plans of mice and men…well, let's just say things don't always work out the way you hoped.

"What's Plan B?" I asked him.

"Mmm, well…I'm sure it'll work out. Don't you think we'll be okay if at least the bedroom and bathroom are finished?"

"And not the kitchen? Not the living room? It's Louisa's first baby, and first labors can take a while. She might appreciate some space to walk around, a little breathing room. If the bedroom is the only completed space downstairs, and the stairs aren't finished, then we'll all have nowhere to hang out except that small bedroom, right?"

"And the bathroom," he answered, as if that solved everything.

"Right. And the bathroom. Is it finished?"

"Everything works except the shower."

I took a deep breath. Bare studs in the bedroom, no insulation, no sheetrock. Bare subflooring. Unfinished windows covered with plywood. Water only in the bathroom sink, but no shower. I tried to imagine a laboring woman, her husband, a midwife and her assistant, and two or three friends all cooped up for hours in this one small, dark, airless room.

I just couldn't see it.

"I really think you might want to consider having the baby at a friend's house," I suggested as gently as possible. "This just doesn't look like it's going to be ready in a month…"

Neither of them replied, so I let it go. It was their birth, not mine.

And of course Louisa's labor started two weeks early. It had rained the day before – again – so the ground around the house was freshly muddy, and the planks laid in lieu of a concrete sidewalk were wobblier than ever. Carrying my supplies, I found the footing especially precarious with a sea of sucking mud threatening to obliterate me at the first misstep.

Beside the front door, Gordon had laid down some large sheets of plywood, and I could see they were intended to function as a sort of patio, an outdoor extension of the minimal livable space inside. A cluster of cheap white plastic chairs sat there, along with a small table, and two of Louisa's friends occupied a couple of the chairs. When they saw me, they came down the plank to help with my gear.

We went inside, and to my eyes, everything looked the same – except the bedroom was insulated, sheetrock was up, and one of the windows was functional. At least we had daylight and fresh air.

"Is the shower working, Gordon?"

"No, no, sorry," he said, without making eye contact. "We've had a few setbacks."

Of course.

Margaret arrived while I was contemplating the situation. She navigated the giant step from the plywood "patio" to the threshold of the front door and stopped in her tracks. I'd told her Louisa would be having her baby "in a house in the middle of a major renovation," but clearly I hadn't been descriptive enough.

She looked left, right, up the "stairway," and then she turned to me.

"…whoa…" she said softly, which I thought showed remarkable restraint.

In the bedroom beyond those dangerous stairs, Louisa paced between the bed and the cardboard boxes that still served as their bureau and closet. She appeared to be entering active labor, but with her two friends, Gordon, Margaret, and me in the room with her, it truly felt claustrophobic. So after I'd checked her condition and the baby's, I suggested we whittle the numbers down to maybe just two. Gordon and one of her girlfriends stayed with Louisa while the rest of us went into the quasi-kitchen.

Margaret looked around. "So…this is the kitchen? I see a brand new Viking stove…does it work?" and she flipped a dial. Nothing. "Right. Not hooked up yet."

I turned on the electric kettle to make tea, and Margaret continued her wandering. "No water. No fridge…" Then she left the kitchen and walked down the hall to the bathroom. When she returned, she said, "No shower, huh?"

I nodded.

She took a deep breath and said, "Okay, then."

Gordon apologized and said they'd been showering at the next door neighbor's house. "She's away on vacation for a week and she said we could continue using her shower while she's gone. I'm assuming that included during the labor, if necessary, although we didn't specifically discuss it."

A few hours later, Louisa began looking stressed. Her demeanor changed, and her soft humming turned to moaning, then became much louder. She peeled off her T-shirt and, without saying a word to anyone she scampered out the door, stark naked. She zipped across the plywood "patio," waded through the mud oozing beneath her feet, and stepped onto her neighbor's lawn. She grabbed a hose, turned on the water, rinsed her feet, and unlocked the back door.

"Why'd she take her clothes off before she went outside?" asked Gordon, understandably puzzled.

"Don't know," I replied. "Given even a little wiggle room, women in labor sometimes do really weird stuff."

Of course, Louisa's friends, her husband, Margaret and I had followed hard on her heels, and when we walked inside, I think we all said, "Aaaah."

Sunlight streamed through starched curtains into a pristine yellow kitchen. A teakettle sat on the stove, and when I turned one of the dials, voila! A steady little gas flame magically appeared. I filled the kettle with water, and soon we all had steaming cups of milky tea in our hands.

Louisa paced down the hallway into the dining room, then turned a corner and headed for the living room. Deep leather chairs and Craftsman lamps with amber mica shades gave the room a serenity that was entirely lacking in her own house. Gordon joined us and watched his wife labor on in her own style: pacing, moaning, swaying, and sometimes singing snatches of an old Simon and Garfunkel song.

One of her friends retrieved a guitar from her car and picked up the melody. Soon we were all singing along to *Hello, lamppost, Whacha knowin'? I've come to watch your flowers growin'...*

No one seemed to know all the words, but we definitely all chimed in with, *doodley-doo-doo, feelin' groovy.*

And, indeed, in that calm, clean, tidy little house, everything felt very groovy.

I'd brought only a Doppler and a blood pressure cuff across the muddy yard, because of course we would be returning to Louisa's house for the birth. After all, that's where my equipment was, and that's where a bedroom was all set up for the birth.

Louisa's moaning became more strident, and at the end of one of her trips back from the living room, she turned away from the kitchen and veered into the bathroom. Margaret and I followed her.

Oh, it was lovely. Two fresh pale green towels hanging from the rack. A white shower curtain with a dark green stripe along the bottom. A pale green throw rug on the floor. Everything else was white tile and white porcelain, except for a small arrangement of dried flowers on the counter and a blue toothbrush.

Louisa climbed into the shower alone. She had let the water pour over her long and very pregnant body for about fifteen minutes when I heard her grunting. I whipped the curtain back, and she was leaning forward with her hands on her knees, clearly pushing. Strands of thick bloody mucus clung to her inner thighs. I took a quick peek, and it was obvious she was about to give birth.

In her neighbor's house.

With no birthing bed prepared, no midwifery equipment, nothing helpful at all, really.

This was *not* the plan.

I said, "Oh, no, no, no. Not here. Get out, Louisa. We have to leave."

"Oh, no, no, no," she said right back to me, and before I could do anything to reinforce my intention to move her outside and into her own bedroom, she leapt from the shower, wrapped one of the pale green towels around her and ran into the bedroom.

Once there, she threw the towel aside and flung herself across what looked like an antique pastel quilt lying, Oh, so beautifully on a brass bed.

"Oh, no, no, no," I said again, but then I peeked between her legs again. The bag of water was bulging, and the baby's dark hair was visible right behind it.

She was minutes from giving birth, in the process of which she would surely destroy her generous neighbor's beautiful quilt, plus the sheets and probably the mattress as well.

I turned to Louisa's two friends and said, "Go get everything. Especially get the plastic off their bed. Hurry," and they dashed out the door. In moments, I saw them returning, arms laden with birthing equipment, an oxygen tank, and a piece of plastic blowing behind them in the wind. When they entered the bedroom, I said, "Louisa, we have to get this plastic under you, or you'll totally trash this lovely quilt."

"No, no, no," she said, and the bag of water bulged out further.

I looked around the room. Margaret, Gordon, Louisa's two friends and I were present, and I thought, Okay, we're going to do this. We absolutely have to.

"On the count of three, everyone grab her and lift her up," and that's what they did. In seconds, Louisa, protesting vocally as she was hoisted into the air, lay on bare plastic…and then her water broke.

And then the baby's head came out.

And then the rest of the baby, and then some blood.

Quite a bit of blood, actually. Followed by more. And even more.

Louisa was hemorrhaging.

I suspected she had abrupted part of her placenta, which would account for the violent speed of late labor and the tumultuous pushing stage.

The placenta is supposed to remain firmly attached to the uterine wall until after the baby's birth. If it begins to separate prematurely, nature's way of trying to save the baby's life is to respond with very rapid labor. That's almost certainly what had happened to Louisa. But because her placenta was only partly separated, the uterus couldn't contract to control bleeding. She would continue bleeding from the exposed blood vessels behind the detached edge of the afterbirth until the rest of it was removed.

The baby, a girl, was fine. But Louisa was still bleeding. Memories of Paula's horrific postpartum hemorrhage just a few months earlier flashed through my mind, and I remember thinking, No, no, no, this can't be happening again.

By then, a pool of blood about two inches deep lay in the hollow between her crotch and her knees, and more spread out the sides and up her back. I put steady traction on the umbilical cord while Margaret called 911. We exchanged glances, and I knew we were both praying different EMTs and paramedics would respond, a different crew from those arrogant and inept guys who had come to Paula's house and delayed transport to the hospital for such a terribly long time.

I rarely ever attempted a manual placenta removal at home for fear of precipitating a hemorrhage. But Louisa was already hemorrhaging, so I decided to go for it, especially as the paramedics were already en route.

It was actually pretty simple, once I started. I closed my fingers around the umbilical cord and slid them up to the point where it inserted into the placenta. As Louisa yelled, "Yow!" I felt for the edge and found where it had come loose. At that point, with my entire hand now inside Louisa's womb, I slipped my fingers behind the loose part and peeled the rest of the placenta away from the uterine wall.

Holding the placenta in my fist, I began removing my hand as

Louisa said, "Whoa, whoa, jeez!" and then, as I withdrew my hand and her placenta entirely, she said, "Ahhhh. Much better. God..."

Then I gave Louisa an injection of Pitocin while Margaret massaged her uterus, which tightened up nicely...and immediately her bleeding stopped. I started an IV with more Pitocin in it to replace some of the fluid volume she'd lost and to help keep her uterus contracted. I let the first third of the bag run in quickly, then adjusted it to a slower drip.

Margaret and I examined the placenta. Sometimes in these cases, the placenta comes away in pieces, and now and then a lobe is left behind. When that happens, bleeding can recur later. But this placenta, as we mounded it up and scrunched it together, appeared intact – no missing parts.

The 911 crew arrived as we were examining the placenta...and what a difference from our last experience.

These guys were polite, respectful, and helpful. I gave them a brief history of the birth and explained why I'd called, although they could certainly see evidence of the hemorrhage with their own eyes. I said I was comfortable with them leaving, as we had things under control by then, but they wanted to take Louisa's blood pressure and sneak a peak at the baby. "Sure, of course," I said, as I was certain they'd have some report they would need to complete at the conclusion of their visit.

Louisa's blood pressure was on the low side, 100/60, but she wasn't dizzy when she sat up to hold the baby, so the guys hung around for about fifteen more minutes, just making small talk, and then they left.

When the first bag of IV fluid was finished, I hung a second bag, and then we began the cleanup. I can't remember ever being so focused, so careful, so thorough. Louisa was surrounded by blood, but none had leaked over the edge of the plastic.

Yet.

Gordon went back to their house and returned with a huge stack of old towels, and we began the slow process of sopping up the blood and carefully transferring the soggy towels into a black plastic trash bag. I was grateful the floor of the bedroom was bare oak, not pale green carpeting, so the few drips that landed on the floor were easily wiped up.

When the puddle of blood was reduced to a minimum, Louisa

rolled to her right side. We washed her back and legs, put a clean towel beneath her – then we repeated the process as she rolled to her left. With a huge towel held tightly between her legs, she sat at the side of the bed for about five minutes; I wanted to make sure she wasn't going to pass out as soon as she rose to her feet.

So far, so good.

Then she stood up, and we all stared at her, ready to lower her back onto the bed – with the plastic still in place, in case she became woozy. She stood still for maybe fifteen seconds, sort of taking stock, thinking, testing her balance. Then she smiled and, holding the towel fore and aft with both hands, toddled into the bathroom.

I removed the green throw rug from the room entirely, as thus far it had escaped any bloodstains. Louisa showered, put another big towel around her body, and returned to her own house. The return trip was far less muddy, as Gordon had repositioned the big sheets of plywood into a wide and dry walkway.

With the utmost care, we rolled up the plastic, folded it into thirds, and slipped it into the garbage bag. I fluffed up the pillows and Margaret straightened the pastel quilt – then we both stood back in amazement. Not a single sign remained of the very bloody birth that had occurred about ninety minutes earlier.

Settled into her own bed in the cluttered bedroom, Louisa nursed her daughter and said, "Olivia. Your name means Life, and I can't wait till you're old enough for me to tell you the story of how your life began."

Four days later, I was at her house for a postpartum visit when the next-door neighbor came over. "Oh, gee, you had the baby. A girl? She was early, huh?"

Louisa said, "Yes, two weeks early, and..."

"Everything go okay?"

"Well, yes, mostly, but..." and together we told the astonished neighbor that her own bed is where Olivia had been born.

'Well, my goodness. Imagine that. You know, when I came home last night, something felt slightly off, but it took me a while to put my finger on it. I always keep the teakettle on the back of the stove, but it was on the front burner when I went to fix my breakfast this morning. I thought that was odd. And when I took my shower, I noticed there was only one towel in the bathroom."

"Oh, sorry, I used the towel – I was in kind of a hurry – but we washed it, and it's on the stairs."

The bemused neighbor returned to her house about fifteen minutes later, smiling, shaking her head, and carrying the spotlessly clean, fluffy pale green towel in her hands.

Another One Called. And Another One

Sometimes it happens in a midwife's practice – a long stretch of no births, and then they all come at once. On a Thursday afternoon, no women in my practice had given birth for the previous ten days. Two women were past their due dates, three were due, and several more had just entered their last three weeks.

Margaret had planned a three-day vacation with her husband and kids, but as time to leave approached, she was reluctant, knowing she would probably miss a birth or two.

"No, you should go," I told her. "It's just for a couple of nights. I know you hate missing births, but there will be plenty as soon as you get back."

So off she went to her vacation home in the tiny village of Inverness, near Point Reyes Station.

And she probably hadn't even crossed the San Rafael Bridge before it began to rain babies. I caught two in the hospital Thursday night. I was still busy with the second of those women when a home birth client called, so I sent Bonnie out to her house to evaluate her. Bonnie called the hospital to let me know it'd be several more hours, so I made it with time to spare…but no sleep.

That baby was born around eleven on Friday morning, and I headed home to bed.

Two hours later, the phone rang, and I drove up into the Oakland hills to catch a woman's third baby. It was fast, and I was looking forward to a good long nap…but just as the mom was climbing out of bed to take a shower, my pager beeped. Alta Bates had just admitted a first-timer of mine.

Kathy Heilig, a nurse and wannabe midwife who had been my helper at the birth (and whose son I'd caught six years earlier), stayed on to watch over the mom and newborn for another couple of hours, and I drove out of the hills back to the hospital in Berkeley's flatlands. It was a long labor, fraught with difficulties, and the tired mom needed lots of help. As she was in the hospital, however, I actually managed to squeeze in a blessed and welcome one-hour nap while Rita, one of the compassionate labor room nurses, took over for me.

That baby finally transitioned from womb to room sometime before lunch on Saturday.

As I pulled into my driveway, tired as a horse ridden hard and put up wet, one of the overdue moms, another first-timer, paged me. I went into my house only long enough to restock my supplies, then up to just north of the university in Berkeley for Jessica's birth...and it took forever. Hard, hard work for all of us. She stalled before she transitioned to late labor. I thought we were going to have to move her to the hospital. However, a weak though regular labor pattern finally reestablished itself, and we all soldiered on. She was so, so tired, and she lay in the bed on her side for a few hours, falling asleep between some of the contractions.

Many midwives who attend home births have perfected the skill of sitting on the floor beside a laboring mom's bed, one hand on her belly, dozing...dozing, then wakening as the uterus tightens under her fingertips in time to talk and reassure and soothe the mom for the duration.

And then falling asleep again.

It's not good sleep. It's not deep or sustained sleep. But it's a heck of a lot better than no sleep at all.

Bonnie arrived after her shift at the hospital, relieved me, and I went into another room and fell sound asleep. At some point, the family dog joined me, and his snoring wakened me. I pushed him off the bed, but he must have crept back up beside me with great stealth, because when Bonnie came to wake me up two hours later, there he was, pressed hard against my back.

Jessica had moved into pushing, but it was still a long and difficult slog. Three hours of hard work finally produced a baby weighing more than nine pounds.

By the time I returned home, it was 7:00 pm on Saturday evening. I had caught what felt like twenty babies since Thursday night, on no more than four hours of interrupted sleep...and one of the overdue moms, Nancy, pregnant with her fifth child, had *not* been among them.

She continued to lurk out there, still great with child.

I downed a bowl of cereal with a banana on top and collapsed in my bed, bones aching with fatigue. And I slept like the dead. Oh, my

God, it felt so good. My own bed, my own pillow, no snoring dog...

And then the phone rang. Tess, two weeks early, was on the line. Her bag of water had broken, and there was meconium in the fluid. I sent her into the hospital, crawled out of bed, took my first shower since Thursday morning, brushed my teeth, and went back to Alta Bates.

Because of the meconium, Tess was attached to a fetal monitor. Her labor began spontaneously, and the baby's heartbeat was mostly okay. But sometimes it got a little wonky, so the rest of the night I stayed with her, keeping an eye on the monitor while walking Tess around the labor room, encouraging her to change position frequently if and when she was in the bed, and talking her through the contractions when they became difficult.

She was progressing, but slowly, slowly. Her temperature was slightly elevated, so it became imperative to get the show on the road. I started an IV, ran a whole bag in quickly to hydrate her, and then connected her to a Pitocin pump when we switched to a second bag.

Finally she kicked into high gear around 3:00 pm.

Tess was an hour into pushing when the labor room nurse called me to the phone. It was my husband.

"Jeez," I said to him. "You must think I left town without telling you. I've caught I don't know how many babies in the past couple of days. But I should be home in maybe two or three hours, and then I'm going to sleep for a week."

"Well, um..."

"What? *What?*"

"Uh, well, there's another one," Rog said, and I could hear the apology in his voice.

"No. No way."

"Yeah, sorry. Someone named Nancy called here at the house, and she's in labor."

"Oh. My. Lord."

I couldn't possibly leave the hospital with Tess pushing, and now I had a woman about to give birth to her fifth baby in El Cerrito, a small town just north of Berkeley.

I called Carole Hagin and Bonnie and asked them to cover for me. Depending on how quickly Tess progressed and how slowly Nancy progressed, perhaps I'd make it. And I really wanted to, because

221

Nancy had never met either Bonnie or Carole.

But things didn't work out that way.

Tess pushed for more than two hours before squeezing out a little six-pounder, and Nancy was in good labor by the time Bonnie arrived.

Bonnie told me later that Nancy was breathing heavily when she arrived, and she knew Carole, who lived nearly an hour away, probably wouldn't make it. She walked into the bedroom where Nancy was kneeling beside the bed and said, "Hi, my name is Bonnie, and I'm going to be your midwife today."

Nancy just laughed and said, "How do you do, Bonnie? I'm glad to meet you."

Nancy had planned to have her other four kids present to welcome this fifth child into the family, but about an hour after Bonnie arrived, just as Nancy was starting to feel pushy, she suddenly said, "I want the kids out."

The kids really wanted to stay, but Nancy was insistent. Becky, the oldest, herded her siblings from the room, but Bonnie was amused to see their four little faces reappear almost immediately outside the bedroom window.

Later, Bonnie told me, "I made sure I didn't block their view, and wow! that baby came out so fast, probably just two contractions later. Then the older kids came tumbling back into the bedroom before I'd even finished drying the baby off. They'd probably been gone not more than five minutes.

"And the six-year-old said, 'Whoa! That was so cool. Just like watching a movie!'"

When I reread their charts later, I realized Tess and Nancy gave birth within six minutes of each other.

Shortly after Tess's birth, I left for Nancy's, and Carole and I arrived within seconds of each other.

Carole said, "Jeez, you look like hell."

"Oh, thank you so much for that, but I'm sure you're right. I've been kind of busy."

I was home by dinnertime on Sunday but far too exhausted to eat a big meal, so my solicitous husband fixed me scrambled eggs, toast, and hot sweet milk.

As I headed upstairs to my bed, the phone rang. My mind screamed, No, no, no, no…but it was Margaret.

"Did I miss any births?"

"Uh, well, yes. Yes, you did."

"Damn. How many?"

I had to think. "Seven," I finally said. "No, wait...eight."

"*Eight?* What?"

"Yep. Everyone who was overdue, everyone who was due, and a couple of early ones. It felt like all the pregnant women in the Bay Area gave birth this weekend. But I'll tell you all about it later. I'm going to bed."

When I woke up sometime before noon on Monday, I gathered the charts and tried to make sense of the numbers. It turned out that, with no more than six hours of fitful sleep, I'd caught seven babies, plus an eighth one that Bonnie went solo on, between 2:00 am on Friday and 5:00 pm on Sunday, a little over sixty hours.

Insane.

And of course not a single birth occurred in the following two weeks. I could have taken a trip to Amsterdam and not missed a thing.

That's midwifery for you.

Bird Bones

Jan was small and thin as a reed. Her long neck, erect posture, and distinctive way of walking made me think she was a ballet dancer. It turned out I was right. She had danced with the San Francisco Ballet for several years but had retired two years earlier in order to start a family.

"I was always watching my weight," she said. "You get paranoid about it, weighing yourself five times a day. I hadn't had a menstrual period for years. I'm pretty sure I wasn't anorexic, because I love to eat – and I *did* eat – but I didn't eat a lot and always made a point of stopping before I was full."

"That's pretty common for professional ballet dancers, isn't it?"

"Very common. And a lot of them are bulimic, too, though I never was. I hate to throw up too much to ever force myself to do it."

"So when you stopped dancing...?"

"Yeah, I put on about fifteen pounds in a year, even though I kept dancing and exercising – but just for pleasure, not as a job anymore. I teach ballet now, but I don't perform publicly."

Looking at her sharp little collarbones showing so prominently beneath the straps of her maternity sundress, I couldn't imagine her weighing fifteen pounds less.

"My periods finally came back, and I was so happy. But then they kept coming, and I wasn't so happy anymore. Each one meant I still wasn't pregnant. Then finally I missed a period...and here we are!"

Her husband, Tommy, was a surgical resident at the University of California San Francisco. He, too, was very thin and appeared to be as athletic as his wife, but he towered more than a foot above Jan's diminutive height. He managed to squeeze a few prenatal visits with her into his busy schedule, and he was proud, with his OB knowledge from medical school, to have a bit more information on the subject than your average first-time expectant dad.

Her pregnancy progressed normally, but her belly was huge. An ultrasound at six months ruled out twins, but as Jan approached term, I wondered if there'd been a mistake. She looked like a beach ball with four limbs and a head attached, but she continued to move like a ballerina – albeit a very rotund ballerina.

Every time she came for a visit, I looked at that big belly and then at her hips, slim as an adolescent boy's, and her thin legs…and I asked myself if it would really be possible for her to give birth vaginally.

Time will tell, I told myself. Time will tell. I'd certainly been surprised before.

A week before her due date, Tommy called me around 2:00 am and sounded pretty excited. "Jan's about to have the baby. She's been having contractions off and on for a couple of hours, so I decided to examine her…and she's fully dilated."

"Really? She's pushing? Can you see the baby?" I cradled the phone between my ear and shoulder as I began preparing for a quick get-away.

"No, not yet. She's pretty calm, actually. I think she's just having a real easy time of it."

Odd, I thought. But I hoped he was right, for Jan's sake. I zipped up into the hills of North Berkeley, fully expecting to be greeted at the door by Tommy with a still-wet baby in his arms. I kept reassuring myself that, as a surgical resident, he would manage things calmly.

But when Tommy opened the door, his arms were empty. Jan, wearing an oversized T-shirt, sat cross-legged on a Chux on a chair in the living room. Her hair was tidy. She looked happy and relaxed, and she was sipping a mug of hot tea.

Weird.

I listened to her belly, and the heartbeat sounded strong and regular. I felt her belly, and soon it hardened and tightened and rounded as bellies do during contractions. "You feeling that?" I asked her.

"Yeah, but really these contractions don't feel much different from all the Braxton-Hicks ones I've been having lately. I can't believe I'm ready to give birth. It's been so easy, nothing like what I was expecting."

"Do you feel pressure, like you want to bear down or push?"

"Nope. I feel just the same as I did yesterday."

Okay, now I had some serious doubts. A surgical resident is not an obstetrician. He's not even an OB resident. Tommy probably hadn't put his hands on a pregnant woman in years.

Maybe, just maybe, Tommy had gotten it wrong.

"May I check you, Jan? I know Tommy just did it half an hour ago, but I want to see for myself."

"Sure," she said. And she hopped off the couch with her usual grace and strolled back to the bedroom where everything had been set up in preparation for the birth.

I checked her.

She most definitely was not fully dilated. She wasn't three centimeters dilated, either. She wasn't even one centimeter dilated.

In fact, she wasn't in labor.

"How much longer will it be?" Tommy asked, and they both looked at me with great expectation.

What to say?

"Well, it could be a while longer. Even a few days, or maybe a week or more.

They both looked shocked.

Tommy swiped his hair back, frowned, and said, "But...wha...?"

"I can understand why you thought Jan was fully dilated, Tommy," I said. "Her cervix is way up high and way toward her back, super posterior and really hard to find. It's all thinned out, and the head is kind of low. I'm pretty sure you were feeling the baby's head through the thin side wall of her cervix."

Tommy was stunned. Then confused. Then embarrassed. He began to fall all over himself apologizing to both of us.

"It's fine, no problem at all," I reassured him, as Jan pulled her panties back on.

Then Tommy poured me a mug of tea. The three of us sat down in the living room, and we had a little chat about the signs of labor, how most women behave during labor, the indications of late labor...all that kind of stuff. We'd been over it all before, but clearly Tommy hadn't been listening. Or perhaps he hadn't truly internalized it. Or possibly thought he already knew all that stuff.

"There *are* such things as silent labors or really easy, virtually painless ones, however. I should know. I had one myself with my second child. But, guys, those labors are rare as hen's teeth. Anyway, I'm sure the next time you call me, Jan will really be in labor."

As I was leaving, I took another look at Jan's tiny little body, nonexistent butt, size five shoes…and I wondered again how likely a home birth really was. I hated to harbor negative thoughts, but she really looked like a walking Cesarean.

Ten days later, Tommy called again, and this time I heard Jan moaning loudly in the background. Okay, this was the real thing.

"She sounds really active, Tommy," I said. "Did you examine her?"

"Oh, *hell*, no! No no no *no!* After last time, I don't trust myself at all. I've just been trying to keep her calm, talking to her, rubbing her back, but gee, she's acting like a tornado just tore the roof off the house."

So I zoomed back up to their house amid the eucalyptus and redwood trees.

I knocked. No answer. I tried the handle, and the door opened, so in I went, and Oh, my! The house was vibrating with birthing energy.

As I entered the bedroom, I could see almost none of Jan at all. Just her big belly, her two skinny legs sticking out on either side, and a ginormous head just a few pushes from birthing. So much head was visible that I really couldn't see Jan's perineum at all. The baby's head took up every bit of space between the bottom of her belly, her thighs, and her bum.

Two contractions after I arrived, I held a screaming ten-pound baby in my bare hands.

Ten pounds. *Ten pounds!*

Before pregnancy, Jan had weighed just a skosh more than one hundred pounds, and although her belly grew to enormous proportions, she'd gained only twenty pounds during the past nine months. Clearly, half of her weight gain had been all baby.

When we'd gathered ourselves together and calmed down from the tumultuous labor, Jan said something that's stayed with me ever since. She said her mother was tiny, too, and all of her babies weighed more than nine pounds. And they'd all been born quickly and easily, delivered by a family practice doctor in a small hospital in Iowa. The doctor had said that, in his experience, women with thin bone structures usually give birth with relative speed and ease. "He said my mom had bird bones," Jan said, "and he believed that women with thin bones are likely to have more space in the pelvis than women with larger, thicker bones."

Bird bones.

I'd never heard the term, but it made a certain sort of contradictory sense...and indeed, in the several decades of my practice, I caught more than a few good-sized babies born to women of diminutive proportions, women with a pelvis that the old-time doctor in Iowa might have diagnosed as being made of "bird bones."

Who am I to argue with that wisdom?

Whatever kind of bone structure Jan had, it had served her well.

Hail Mary

When I was in third and fourth grade, I lived on the second floor of an apartment building in Chicago, Illinois. Across the street lived Renée Yocherer, who quickly became my best friend.

Her family originally came from Strasbourg, a city in a region that has been bounced back and forth between France and Germany for centuries, depending on the vagaries of war. When France was occupied by Germany in 1940, Strasbourg was annexed to Germany. After liberation in 1944, the region was returned to France.

Renée's father considered himself German, and he pronounced his last name as if it were spelled "Yocker." Renée's mother pronounced the same name "Yosheray," accent on the last syllable, giving it a decidedly French twist.

When her father wasn't around, they spoke French at home, which utterly charmed me, but as soon as he came home from work each day, they switched to English or German.

While her father scorned all religion, Renée's mother was a devout Catholic, and their children were raised in her faith. It was my first introduction into how different her religious life was when compared to my Protestant upbringing in the Episcopal church.

Renée always wore a scapular of the Sacred Heart of Jesus either pinned to her cotton undershirt or on a string around her neck, beneath her clothing and touching her skin. Candles flickered in front of religious statues sitting on tables in nearly every room of their apartment. Of course, she attended Catholic school and was taught by nuns with rosaries dangling from belts around their voluminous habits.

While I went to school five days a week, it seemed Renée was home from school about once every three weeks. "It's Saint So-and-So's Day," she explained, "so we just go to church in the morning, and then we have the rest of the day off.

Sometimes on these frequent saints' days, out of sheer boredom – and probably also out of curiosity – she came to school with me. But I never got to go to school with her, of course, because I attended public school and they definitely didn't send us home just because it was St. Somebody's Day.

Renée and her family didn't eat meat on Fridays. When she told me this, I was speechless. It was the early Fifties, a staunch meat and potatoes era, and I couldn't conceive of a family dinner that didn't include meat.

"But what do you eat, then?" I asked.

"Tuna casserole or frozen fish sticks, usually," she said. "Sometimes grilled cheese sandwiches with tomatoes and pickles in them."

It was those Fridays that gave me an opportunity to get an inside peek into her religious life. When I came home from school, she was waiting for me, and we walked together to St. Margaret's, the parish church attached to her school.

I sat in a pew while she made her confession. As she stood in a line of similarly-aged children waiting their turn, I wondered what these little Midwestern girls with bows in their hair and boys with skinned knees could possibly have done that would warrant kneeling in front of a priest and reeling off a list of sins.

"What did you confess?" I asked her. I was insatiably curious as she returned from the darkness of the mysterious confessional to sit beside me in the pew. I wondered if it was forbidden for her to tell me, like you mustn't tell what you wish for when you blow out birthday candles – or the wish won't come true. Maybe it was a sin if she told me what she'd told the priest. I just didn't know if it was okay, but I *definitely* wanted her to tell me.

No problem. Renée began ticking off her sins on her fingers. "Oh, let's see. This week I told the priest I stuck gum under my desk, I sassed my mother, and I lied to the nuns two times. I think that's all. Sometimes I have to make stuff up, because otherwise they'll think I'm hiding something. I can always say I was mean to my brother, though, because I usually am."

"Then what? Why do you always pray afterwards?"

"The priest, he gives us a penance to 'atone for our sins.' I don't really know what that means, but today I just have to say ten Hail Marys. He's the nice priest."

She knelt, held her rosary between her fingers, and began rapidly slipping around the beaded circle, muttering under her breath. After crossing herself, she stood up, tucked the rosary into her pocket, and we walked out of the dim church that smelled of dust, old flowers, and candle wax.

"What are those beads for?" I asked.

"They're to help count the prayers. We've got a bunch of Hail Marys and Our Fathers, the Gloria, and then Salve Regina comes at the end."

"Wha…?" The Our Father, okay, I knew that was what we called The Lord's Prayer in the church I went to, but the other stuff? She might as well have been speaking Hindi.

So she taught the prayers to me, and when we spent the night at each other's house, which was often, we prayed her prayers and then my prayers. Soon they came easily to my lips, including the rather pitiful Salve Regina with its "poor banished children of Eve" and all the "mourning and weeping in this valley of tears." But there was something seductive about the cadence of the language, and I've never forgotten those words I learned in childhood.

However, I certainly never thought I would be called on to recite them to laboring women.

Especially Jewish women.

* * *

The first was Ellie, a young Jewish woman married to an Irish Catholic. Ellie's labor was long and arduous, and as she finally drew near the end, with the contractions piling on hard and fast, she began chanting, "Holy Mother of God," and "Jesus, Mary, and Joseph," and "Sweet Jesus on the cross," over and over during each one.

Her mother, knitting in the corner while keeping an eye on a large pot of chicken soup simmering on the stove, was utterly and frankly appalled.

"Ellie, Ellie, what is that you're saying? You talking to Jesus, now? And Mary? Like, the Virgin Mary? What is going on here?"

Ellie ignored her, and with the next contraction she began reciting snatches of the Hail Mary prayer. Her husband chimed in, and soon I was right in there with them – the three of us saying Hail Marys like a repeating rosary loop during each of her contractions.

"Ellie, Ellie, Ellie! My child! So what is this?" said her mother, and I really felt sorry for the woman. "What is this *meshuga* stuff

233

you're saying? I raised you to be a good Jewish girl."

"Ma, shut up, just shut up!" and her mother's eyes popped wide open. "Ma, I'm sorry, I'm sorry, but it's stuff I've heard David saying. I don't know why, Ma, I really don't, but it's working. So leave me alone, okay?"

Ellie's mother didn't say another word, but every time I looked at her, she was biting her lips between her teeth, surely trying to prevent herself from unleashing a torrent of protest.

Whether it was the walking, the four showers Ellie took, or the hundreds of Hail Marys uttered during the following hours, something worked, and Ellie's baby boy was finally born.

When the baby was handed to her, Ellie's mother bundled the child into her arms, turned her back on the rest of us, and began speaking rapidly to him in a low voice.

I can only imagine what she was saying.

* * *

The second woman was Marion, pregnant with her first baby at age forty. She had used artificial insemination to conceive and intended to bring up her child as a single mom. She was a professional woman of significant financial means, and she had employed Jeanette, a young woman from Quebec, to be a full-time nanny.

Jeanette came to live with Marion a month before the baby was due, because Marion wanted them to get to know each other well. She also wanted the younger woman to be thoroughly familiar with the house, the kitchen, the neighborhood, the stores – just everything, really, so the transition would go smoothly when Marion returned to work three months after giving birth.

Marion's identity as a Jew was more cultural than religious, she had told me, which is not uncommon. I doubt the question of religion had ever come up when she was interviewing women for the nanny job, however, because it just wasn't that important to her.

Marion had a cluster of women friends at her birth, most of them professionals, and only two had had children. The four or five childless women present during the labor appeared awestruck – perhaps a little overwhelmed, maybe even fearful – at the raw power of the occasion. Those who had given birth themselves drew close to Marion, stroked her, whispered to her, and supported her as she walked around the house.

But the others, along with Jeanette, stayed mostly on the periphery...and then I saw Jeanette's lips moving soundlessly. I suspected she was praying.

Marion, like many women, steadily shed her clothing as she progressed through her long labor until eventually she was naked. During one of her circuits through the house, she took a right turn and headed into the bathroom.

"You want to try the shower?" I asked.

"No, the tub," said Marion, and she turned on the water.

Birth is primal, and so is water. Earth, Air, Fire, and Water, the basic elements of life. A laboring woman is grounded to the earth, is often pulled soaring into the air, inevitably feels the heat of the fire... but water is the element that seems most powerful during birth. Once introduced to streams of water running over their heads and faces, their bodies, backs, and bellies, many women never want to leave the shower.

"It just feels right," countless women have told me, sighing with relief.

The same goes for a tub of water. But the effect of a warm bath on a woman's labor can be very different from that of a shower. The tub sometimes relaxes a woman so effectively that eventually we must haul her onto dry land to get the process moving again.

A tub can slow a labor down, but a shower rarely does.

Fortunately, Marion's contractions continued at a steady clip while she lay in the bathtub. And she developed an interesting routine. She had filled the tub nearly to the brim, and with each contraction she submerged herself, including her whole head, until only the highest part of her belly rose above the waterline. She rarely came up for air more than twice during her contractions, which were lasting a minute or more, and as I watched a slow stream of small bubbles rise from her nose and mouth, I was mightily impressed with her lung capacity and breath-holding ability.

Between contractions, she pushed herself up until her head and chest were out of the water – and then she noticed Jeanette's lips moving.

"What are you doing?" she asked, and everyone turned to look at the young woman.

Jeanette looked mortified. "Nothing," she mumbled.

"Are you praying?"

"Kind of," she said, looking as though she wanted the earth to swallow her.

"What are you praying?"

"Uh, I'll stop. Do you want me to leave? I can go," and she edged toward the door.

"No, no. I want to know what you're saying."

"It's the Hail Mary prayer."

"Can you say it out loud? I want to hear it."

Before Jeanette could start, however, another contraction began. Marion closed her eyes and went underwater again. I suspect being beneath the warm water was a form of sensory deprivation, absence of sounds, sights, all distractions, and it seemed to allow Marion to just *Be*. She was in her own space, all alone with her labor.

When the contraction ended, she rose slowly, looked at Jeanette, and said, "Okay, say it now."

And Jeanette did. "Hail Mary, full of grace, the Lord is with thee. Blessed art thou among women…"

"Yeah, yeah. I like that. Just keep saying it. Does anyone else know that prayer?"

Heads shook No – except for mine and one other woman's.

"Go for it, then. And don't stop. It's working for me."

So for the two hours remaining until Marion reached full dilation, three of us recited the Hail Mary endlessly in the gaps between contractions. During pushing, however, Marion wanted no part of the prayer. She was in an entirely different mental space and needed energy, not contemplation.

When she finally held the baby in her arms, she looked at me and said, "I'll bet that's the first time a Jewish woman has asked you to say the Hail Mary during her labor."

"Actually, no," I said, and I told her about Ellie.

Seahorse in the Caul

Smack.

No, not quite *smack*; more of a soft *splat* or very muted clap.

Not a loud sound, but arresting. Definitely arresting, and entirely out of place.

With the kitchen phone in my hand and Bonnie's number half-dialed, I paused, listening...and I heard nothing.

But what had that odd sound been? I punched in the last few digits, then stuck my head around the door to look at Nancy, hunkering near the floor and supported from behind by Gretchen, her partner.

Nancy looked at me, her face mirroring what I imagined was my own puzzled expression.

Splat?

"What was that?" she asked.

"Yeah. Weird sound. What was it?" Gretchen asked.

* * *

I had arrived at Nancy and Gretchen's house only forty minutes earlier in what we all assumed to be the beginning of active labor. However, when I examined Nancy, her cervix dilated from four to seven centimeters during a single contraction, and I knew she would be delivering very, very quickly, perhaps before Bonnie had a chance to come assist me.

Having decided on a home birth only a week earlier, Nancy and Gretchen had minimal prep time and were unprepared when labor began just five days later, three weeks before the due date. Nancy's cousin, Tim, had arrived to help out and was bustling around the bedroom in a flurry of activity. With the birth bed unmade, no supplies organized, the post-birth celebratory lasagna unthawed, and Nancy's baby heading Earthside with the speed of a toddler on a sliding board, Tim had his work cut out for him.

Nancy and Gretchen moved into the dining room to get out of his way.

Then, like an interrupted hiccup, Nancy's breath caught at the back of her throat and she dropped into a squat.

Glancing at the Oriental carpet, I thought, Uh-oh, blood, amniotic fluid, and birth goop. I yanked the carpet back and pulled Gretchen onto a dining room chair. Nancy moved over and squatted between Gretchen's spread thighs, her bare bottom almost touching the polished oak floor.

So there I was, holding a ringing phone, wondering what that odd sound could have been. There is just no proper place in childbirth for exactly that sound.

* * *

Nancy and Gretchen were still looking at me, waiting for an explanation.

Hedging, I said, "I'm not sure. Tim, come here, please, and hold the phone. I need to check something...."

Gazing over his shoulder at the still unmade bed, Tim hurried toward me, dragging a plastic mattress cover behind him.

"When Bonnie answers, tell her to come," I said, leaving him standing there with the receiver in his hand, looking as puzzled as the rest of us.

Now Nancy's eyes followed me as I hurried toward her. Two little frown lines appeared between her eyebrows. "I think something might have slipped out. Kind of. Maybe."

I looked down and blinked.

My thoughts spun like the rotating cherries and grapes in the windows of a Las Vegas slot machine. It took only a split second, but in the moments before cherries appeared in all the windows, I wanted most of all to shout for the world to stop long enough for me to find a camera. I needed time to record something I had not thought possible. Something way beyond inconceivable. Something far off into the realm of the utterly impossible.

On the floor between Nancy's feet and under the curve of her belly lay the intact bag of water with the baby bobbing around inside. She had been born "in the caul," the term used to describe a birth in which the baby is expelled while still inside the intact amniotic sac.

Although I'd seen it a few times, it's a rare and magical event...

But there was more, something I'd never read about or even heard of. Still adhering to the outside of the intact bag was the placenta, spread like a benevolent hand cupping the miracle within. The entire contents of the uterus had been expelled, more or less effortlessly to judge from Nancy's look of mere curiosity.

It lay there before me, still jiggling, a transparent water balloon with a baby inside and a placenta attached to the outside...lying intact in a ridiculously small puddle of blood.

Nancy didn't know she'd given birth. That was amazing enough. But equally amazing was the baby, who didn't yet know she'd been born.

Like a dreamy seahorse drifting alongside a strand of kelp, the baby – eyes closed and body curled – floated beside her umbilical cord. Both the baby and the cord still wobbled from the sudden drop to the floorboards a few inches below Nancy's buttocks.

Far more than surprised, I was awestruck at the miracle I was privileged to see, and I wanted to drink in the whole scene, take time to appreciate the once-in-a-lifetime opportunity to which I was an astonished witness.

But, no. I knew what had happened, what must have happened, so I couldn't take time to appreciate what my eyes were seeing because, potentially, I had a life-threatening complication on my hands.

The baby, entirely contained in the sac, very still and quite small, appeared to be sleeping.

Or dead.

Dead was a distinct possibility.

Only a complete placental abruption – the placenta sheering off from the uterine wall before the baby's birth, instead of afterward, as it is supposed to – could have created this scenario. And complete abruptions are always, according to the textbooks, according to my experience, according to every bit of obstetrical and midwifery wisdom I'd ever heard, always accompanied by catastrophic blood loss, profoundly distressed – or dead – babies, and mothers heading rapidly into severe shock.

But here was a puddle of blood that wouldn't have filled a glass holding a medium latté, and Nancy, pink-cheeked and slightly disheveled, looked only puzzled. Definitely not going into shock.

And the baby really did appear to be asleep, curled into a tuck like a drowsy newborn in a Snugli. Not flaccid and floppy. Not dead.

Just sleeping.

What I was looking at existed only in the abstract. It was as if, in a cut-away drawing from an OB textbook, the images of muscles and bones had been peeled away to show how everything was situated within the mysterious interior world of a pregnant uterus. It was an image that lived only on paper, not in real life. But here that image was, in all its glistening, shimmering, and trembling innocence, lying on the hardwood floor in front of me.

Completely, purely, and utterly impossible. Yet there it was.

As these thoughts whirled in my head, I knelt and scooped the whole package into both palms, not daring to lift it too far off the floor because it was so tippy, so bobbley-rolly-jiggly, that I knew it might easily slip out of my hands and drop to the floor again.

It might even roll away from me.

Exactly like a slick, wet, under-inflated water balloon, it gave me no purchase, no handle, no point at which I could get a good grip. And of course my birth supplies, my instruments with sharp things I could have used to rupture the tough bag of water, lay in the bedroom beyond my reach.

I squeezed the water sac, trying to break it. I clawed it. I tried grabbing a bit of the sac and pinching it, twisting it. Nothing was working.

"What *is* that?" asked Nancy.

I'd completely forgotten Nancy and Gretchen.

"It's the baby," I mumbled, "and she's still in the water bag, and I'm trying to…"

"The *baby?*" Nancy and Gretchen squealed in unison.

Nancy looked dumbfounded, and I didn't blame her. "Wait. It's *out?* When did *that* happen? But…is that the *baby?*"

And I realized what I held in my hands, what they were now both looking at, certainly didn't look like the baby they'd been expecting.

Tim called from the doorway. "Bonnie just answered, and she wants to know what's happening."

"Um, wait a sec."

Think, Peggy, think, and hurry up. The baby was born, but so was the placenta. Fortunately, the baby had been separated from her blood supply for only a very short time, but at any moment she'd begin to feel the effects of the lack of oxygen in her blood stream, and she would try to breathe.

I had to free her from this water bag. Just as I was seriously considering mashing my face against the sac and biting it, I had another idea.

I gently laid the whole bundle on the floor, and with one hand I stretched the bag taut over the infant's face. With my pinky finger, I pushed between her lips, into her mouth, past her tongue...

It seemed as though I was halfway down her throat. Would this sac never break? Would I really have to bite it?

Even though I was expecting it, hoping for it, praying for it, when the bag finally burst with a geyser of warm water, it startled me enough to make me yelp. Nancy and Gretchen yelped, too.

....and there was the baby lying in my hands with the remnants of the amniotic sac hanging down like a bridal veil. The startled baby flung her arms and legs out, opened her eyes wide...and she screamed.

"Oh, wow, it *is* the baby." Gretchen's voice was barely audible above the caterwauling infant.

"What? What's happening?" Tim asked.

"Oh, Timmy, the baby's already here." Nancy reached toward her naked, wet, and furious daughter.

"But, how...?"

"I can't really explain it to you right now," I muttered, placing the baby in Nancy's arms. I grabbed a flowered placemat and two cloth napkins from the dining room table to dry her off.

Tim spoke into the phone. "What? Oh, I don't know. I'll ask her." He turned to me. "Um, Bonnie says she can hear the baby crying. Do you still want her to come?"

I breathed in, exhaled slowly, and looked around.

Nancy was fine, crooning to her daughter. The baby was fine: small, for sure, just probably a bit under six pounds, but feisty as the dickens, shaking her fists in the air and turning all beautiful shades of purple and red and pink. Gretchen and Tim were fine, too, although speechless and dazed.

And finally, I was fine, too.

Really, everything was just fine. Without a strong need for Bonnie's assistance any longer, I could think of no real reason for her to make the trip across town.

I turned to Tim and said, "Yes."

Tim blinked. "Yes? Yes what?"

241

"Yes. I want Bonnie to come."

"You do? You want her to come?"

"Yes. Yes I do. I need her to…Um, I just need her to come listen to me."

Tim gave me a strange look, then shrugged and spoke into the phone. "Yeah, she says she needs you to come listen to her…I don't know, that's just what she said."

When Bonnie arrived, she helped me get everyone settled into the bedroom that Tim had finally finished organizing. We fixed a pot of tea, opened a cookie tin where we found the best homemade almond macaroons I've ever eaten, and the two of us sat down facing each other.

"Okay. What?" Bonnie asked.

"You're not going to believe this," I said. "I don't even know if I'll be able to explain it so you'll understand, but I just needed you here. I need to talk to someone who can appreciate how totally bizarre, how completely impossible and weird this birth was. Listen."

And I had the satisfaction of watching her already huge brown eyes get bigger and bigger and bigger as I talked.

Abbey Again

Abbey was pregnant with her second baby. She is the mom for whom I'd flown from California to New York City in March 2014, with hopes of catching her first baby in her studio apartment in the NYU Law School dorm.

Her first pregnancy had been hyper-planned...and, improbably, everything played out exactly according to her script.

"I'm going to give birth on the 14th," she'd said, "because that's the first day of spring break, and I'll have a whole week before I have to go back to class."

"Okay..." I murmured, thinking, Yeah, of course you will.

Not.

"And I haven't asked anyone's permission to have the baby in the dorm because I don't want them to have the opportunity to say No. So I haven't told anyone I'm having it here...well, except for our friends next door, just in case."

Actually, 1 completely agreed with her on this aspect of her planning. In my opinion, it's usually best to go ahead with your plans, whatever they are, assuming it will be okay with "the authorities," ... and then apologize later if it turns out you were wrong.

"And I don't want anyone to come storming in while I'm in labor and try to make me leave. So I'm not going to make any noise. None at all."

I remember smiling to myself, bemused by her supreme self-confidence. While I thought the odds of her giving birth in the dorm were excellent, I gave her chances of having the baby on the 14th and making absolutely no noise during labor exactly equal to the chance of a snowball in hell.

Covering all my bases, I booked a ticket that spanned three weeks.

I should have believed her.

Abbey's first baby, Nico, was born on the 14th. Not only was he born on the 14th, but he was born at 12:20 am on that date, using up only twenty minutes of the 14th and therefore giving her another whole day before classes would resume.

And she didn't make a sound.

She cried softly toward the end of transition, and she whispered, "This fucking hurts" once, but otherwise she silently got out of the way as her uterus, all under its own power, very rapidly pushed her son into the world.

Really.

Her birth story, "The Baby of a Baby," is the final chapter in my previous book, *Midwife: A Calling* (Ant Press, 2015).

So, given her track record for "organization," I wasn't even slightly surprised when she got pregnant within a couple of months of planning for the conception of her second baby. She and her husband, EZ, had moved back to the Bay Area just a week after her graduation, so at least this time I wouldn't have to travel three thousand miles to attend the birth. In fact, they rented a house that my husband and I own, and it is only ten minutes from where we live.

But there was a little confusion about exactly when conception had occurred. Her menstrual history, her early signs of pregnancy, a couple of early ultrasounds, and the onset of her predictably nasty morning sickness gave mixed messages…so she ended up with a due date of November 30, with a little wiggle room on each end.

As my California midwifery license has lapsed and I am officially retired, Abbey found a group of local midwives she felt comfortable with, just in case problems arose. I met them twice at her home before the end of the pregnancy, and they were way groovier than the New York midwife who had attended her first birth. These women were California midwives of the crunchy granola type, in the best sense of the word.

Thanksgiving came and went, and I became anxious because I was scheduled to speak at a birth-related workshop in San Francisco on the December 2nd. A trip to the City can take anywhere from twenty minutes to an hour or more, depending on traffic.

That night, I walked into a room with about twenty women – doulas, midwives, and pregnant moms. They greeted me, and I settled myself into a chair, saying, "I'm so very happy I made it here, because, while I'm not actively practicing midwifery any more, I'm going to be catching the second baby of a dear friend any day now. She went very quickly with her first baby, so I'm…"

...and my cell phone rang.

I glanced down. It was Abbey.

I looked up at the eager, upturned faces of my audience and said, "You're not going to believe this."

They burst out laughing as I said, 'Hello, Abbey. What's up?"

She was having regular contractions, but they were still around ten minutes apart. However, she'd had such a rapid and efficient labor followed by an almost non-existent second stage that I knew I needed to get back across the Bay Bridge and into Oakland as quickly as possible.

My husband had dropped me off with plans to return in several hours, so I was without a car.

I said, "This is crazy, but I need a ride."

Ruthie Davis, one of the co-sponsors of the group, quickly offered. While she gathered my belongings and left to pull her car up close to the storefront where we were meeting, I spoke at triple speed to this understanding bunch of ladies. I read a very short chapter from my last book, signed perhaps a dozen copies ...and I was gone.

When I got home, I called Abbey.

"They're still about ten, sometimes fifteen, minutes apart. Not really very strong, though."

"Do you think you could sleep?"

"Maybe. I don't know. I could try."

I feel it's best to try, as long as possible during labor, to stay on a regular day/night rhythm. As a midwife, I was loath to try to stimulate a woman's contraction pattern during the night, unless, of course, there was some overriding reason to do so. So I generally encouraged women in early labor to sleep or at least rest as much as possible until morning.

With daybreak, birds waken, shake their feathers, and get on with the business of living their busy lives. Women in a desultory labor pattern react much the same way: they waken, they shower, brush their teeth and get their energy flowing, perhaps they have a little breakfast...and they move on with the business of birth.

So I encouraged Abbey to go to bed as if nothing were happening, and I went to bed myself.

All night, I kept telling myself, Sleep, Peggy, sleep. She's only ten minutes away. That's only three contractions worth of mileage. You'll get there, you'll get there...but I kept tossing, rolling over, and checking the clock.

Turns out she'd slept pretty well – definitely better than I did – wakening only a few times with mild contractions. Quite certain labor would kick in for real as soon as she became active, she called Charlotte, her mom, just after sunrise to come pick up Nico, an early riser.

She waited a while until she was pretty sure her mom would be on her way, and then she got out of bed...and immediately the contractions became stronger.

EZ dressed Nico and at 7:00 am, Charlotte took him back to her house in North Berkeley. Then Abbey called me.

Primed, wired, and waiting, it took me only a few minutes to get out the door, and I was at her house half an hour later.

She was definitely in labor. Her midwives had been concerned about making it in time, but two of them lived fairly close by, so they arrived around 8:15. One listened to the baby's heartbeat while the other set out a few supplies in the bedroom.

By 9:00 am, I recognized the signs of late labor when Abbey began resting her head on EZ's shoulder and crying softly during the contractions. She was fully clothed, including leggings, and she was standing in the dining room. I stood beside her, stroked her hair and her back in rhythm with her breathing, whispered into her ear...and expected her to quickly launch into the same almost explosive pushing phase she had experienced with Nico's birth. I was fully prepared to see her drop to the floor any second, and I anticipated pulling down her leggings and catching Baby Nora before Abbey's pants even reached her knees.

But it didn't happen that way. The hard part that comes before pushing didn't change, and it seemed to me something was holding things up.

I knew from talking earlier with her midwives that they do very few vaginal exams during labor. One had said, "We almost never check a woman who's had a baby before."

Officially, they were in charge. As a courtesy, they were allowing me to catch the baby. It felt a little awkward, because I wanted to check her and see if I could help her get past whatever was preventing her from reaching the end of this phase. But I didn't want to step on anyone's toes.

I thought about it for a couple of minutes, and then I did the obvious: I decided to let Abbey make the decision.

I said, "It feels to me like you're close to having the baby, but something seems to be holding things up. Would you like me to check you?"

She nodded, and without a word she hurried down the hall to the bedroom, peeled off her leggings and panties, and lay on the bed. EZ, wordlessly strong, supportive, and loving, sat beside her and held his arm around her.

I checked her between contractions and found her almost fully dilated – but the cervix was way, way, *way* posterior. Instead of being lined up on the same plane as the vaginal canal, it literally was at right angles to the vagina, and the opening was aimed at her spine.

The force of the contractions was pushing the baby against the side of the cervix instead of toward the opening. And the bag of water was still intact.

"Abbey, your cervix is tilted toward the back."

"Is that bad?"

"No, but it'll take a while longer."

"How much longer?" she asked, silent tears running down her cheeks.

"I don't know. A while. But I can make it happen more quickly, if you like."

"How?"

"I could break the bag of water and then pull the cervix forward, if you want me to. Then I'd hold it there during the next contraction. It'll hurt when I pull it forward and hold it in place, but the baby will come out."

"How soon?"

"No guarantee, but considering Nico's birth, I'd say not more than one or two contractions."

She glanced at EZ, then looked back at me and nodded. "I'm ready."

I turned to the two quiet midwives behind me, and one of them already had an Amnihook, a long plastic "crochet hook," in her hand. I took it, inserted it and guided it way around to the back, and I snagged the membrane.

About half a cup of clear amniotic fluid trickled out as I held onto the edge of Abbey's cervix with two fingers and slowly pulled it forward. Abbey whimpered and tensed, but then another contraction began.

I pulled the cervix all the way to the front...and then it melted away completely...and the baby's head was visible. Abbey pushed involuntarily through the end of that contraction.

With the next one, the baby's head crowned, and I was able to guide it the rest of the way out between contractions. As the shoulders rapidly appeared, one of EZ's hands came down, and he helped me curl the onrushing baby onto Abbey's belly and into her arms.

Nora was born at 9:26 am. Pushing had taken less than five minutes.

No more tears. Abbey and EZ admired their daughter as she took her first breath and filled the room with the sounds of a healthy newborn.

* * *

While Abbey was showering, EZ called Charlotte and asked her to bring Nico back home.

"But, wait. What? The baby's born already? We just barely got here."

Instead of Nico first meeting his sister while she was being held by his mother, EZ and Abbey's plan was to place the baby in her crib and introduce Nico to her more independently.

Nico and Charlotte arrived half an hour later, and EZ played with his son for a few minutes in the front of the house. Then Abbey came into the room, kissed Nico, and said, "Baby Nora is here, Nico. Shall we go see her?"

Nico looked puzzled, then smiled and nodded. EZ picked him up, and the three of them walked into the back bedroom, now Nora's room.

Dressed all in white, wearing a white cap, and wrapped in a soft hand-knitted blanket, there lay Nora. Abbey picked her up and sat on the single bed on the far side of the room. Nico sat on EZ's knee and stared at the baby. He looked at Abbey, and then he turned and looked at his father... then back at the baby.

A big smile spread over his face, and he pointed to her.

"It's your sister, Nico. It's Nora. Her name is Nora."

He leaned forward and very, very gently fluttering his lashes, he gave her kisses on her cheeks and eyelids.

Butterfly kisses.

If you enjoyed *Midwife: A Journey*, please
consider leaving a review. Thank you!

Excerpt from the next book in the series

MIDWIFE: AN ADVENTURE

You Can't Make Me

Vanessa didn't have time to get prenatal care. In fact, she didn't have time to have a baby. Vanessa was a very busy woman.

She owned and managed a popular organic food store and sandwich shop on Berkeley's iconic Telegraph Avenue, and one of her best employees was Matt.

Matt graduated from UC Berkeley, then went to law school at Stanford. Hired immediately by one of San Francisco's many prestigious law firms, he quickly realized that being a successful lawyer was far more than a full-time job. He didn't have time to go windsurfing on the bay. He didn't have time to bake sourdough bread with the starter his mother had given him years earlier. He didn't have time to hike in the Berkeley Hills or among the mysterious and sacred redwood trees in Muir Woods. With piles of legal briefs and law books taking up floor space in his high-rise San Francisco condo, he didn't have time for reading the literary nonfiction books that were his preference.

So, giving only ten days notice, he quit.

Everyone told him he was nuts.

"What will you do for money?"

"How will you afford your condo payments?"

"Are you crazy? You're on track to be a partner in a couple of years and you're just…quitting?"

In truth, Matt did kind of wonder how he would support himself. For starters, he sold his condo and moved into a studio apartment in Berkeley, a location he preferred to San Francisco anyway. "Better weather, more interesting people, and less crowded," he later told me, "and way less expensive." He sold his Jaguar and bought a good bike.

And Vanessa hired him to work behind the deli counter at her store, making sandwiches.

Matt helped her close up after the last customer left in late afternoon, and they fell into an easy routine. He put away the food needing refrigeration while she checked stock; he scrubbed the meat counter while she swept; he counted the money while she took a sandwich to the homeless guy in the alley; he set the alarm while she grabbed her purse...and they walked out together, locking the door and pulling down the metal gate behind them.

Before long, he moved in with her...and then she thought maybe she'd missed her period. Probably not, but...maybe. She really hadn't been paying attention.

But remember: Vanessa was a very busy woman. A single mom with sole support of two teenage sons in high school, she was barely managing to keep up with payments on her small two-bedroom house in Albany. Her twelve-year-old car was paid off, she bought her skirts and tops at one of Berkeley's many funky used-clothing stores, and her kids had after-school jobs, but still...she felt she always teetered on the edge.

So she did what many women do when caught by an unexpected (and truth be told, unwanted) pregnancy.

She ignored it.

Matt noticed her belly. Probably raised his eyebrows.

Vanessa probably frowned and shook her head. Or waved off his questions.

Eventually, perhaps about the time she began to leave her shirts hanging loose instead of tucking them into the waistband of her elastic-waisted hippie throwback paisley skirts, denial ceased to work.

She was well and truly pregnant, and there was no getting around the fact. So she came to me.

She was late for her first appointment, of course, as she was late for every single subsequent appointment. Lots of excuses: Too busy, I forgot, the car wouldn't start, Matt didn't remind me, lots of customers...

Too busy, too busy, too busy.

In spite of the chaos she caused with my efforts to keep clinic hours flowing smoothly, I couldn't help but like her. She was funny, sarcastic, and fatalistic. And with pale freckled skin, unruly curls of red hair tumbling over her shoulders, and her fairy wood-sprite wardrobe, she looked glorious as the pregnancy thickened her torso.

"When was your last period?" I had asked at her first visit.

"Not a clue," she said. "I've been too busy to pay attention. No. Wait. I had a period between Halloween and I think Thanksgiving."

"Between the end of October and the third week of November?"

"Maybe."

This was years before ultrasounds were so ubiquitous, and I certainly didn't put women at risk by doing an x-ray for the purpose of establishing a due date. So I resorted to the appearance of other pregnancy symptoms to try to nail down a range for a likely due date.

"Did you get nausea, morning sickness?"

"Hmm, maybe a little. I just thought it was stress."

"Do you remember when it began?"

"Nope. Well, it was after Christmas…and probably before Easter. Yeah, probably…"

"Have you felt the baby move?"

"Oh, sure. That's when I could no longer pretend this wasn't happening. The absolutely last thing I need in my life right now is another child, let alone a baby. I mean, a baby? I don't have time to make a proper dinner most nights for the two hungry kids I've already got, but a baby? Jesus, Mary, and Joseph."

Trying to pull her back to the business at hand – figuring out when this surprise baby was due – I asked, "Do you remember when you felt the first kicking?"

"Oh, sometime after Easter. Maybe. Yeah, I remember the daffodils were blooming. Or was it the day lilies?"

Berkeley is a city of microclimates. Native California orange poppies in one neighborhood bloom four to six weeks ahead of poppies in another neighborhood. Looking as though they've been splashed with black-raspberry ice cream, the plum trees on my sunny urban street burst into bloom a full month ahead of my friend's tree up in the shadier hills.

Really, trying to date a pregnancy based on which flowers were in bloom when Vanessa had noticed the first kicks was nuts. Besides, I strongly suspected she'd actually felt movement weeks earlier but had still been in denial.

A woman pregnant with her first child usually feels the kicks around the twentieth week. That same woman may feel her second baby move two or four weeks earlier – but not because of anything to do with the baby. It's just that once a woman has felt those distinctive flutters, she never forgets, and she recognizes them for what they really are quite a bit earlier second time around.

But Vanessa had been too busy to pay attention.

So, while this was her third pregnancy, she was entirely vague about all of her symptoms. She had just been too distracted, too shocked, and too freaked out to pay attention.

I remember thinking a Ouija board or Tarot cards might be useful. But I measured her belly, grabbed a calendar and played around with her poorly-remembered dates of the landmarks of pregnancy. Somehow I came up with a range of six weeks. She wanted a home birth, so we agreed that if labor started within that period of time, I'd catch her baby at home. But if the baby came more than a week ahead of my fluid "prediction," she would go into the hospital.

During Vanessa's prenatal visits, she left Matt at the shop to hold down the fort, so I didn't meet him until much later in her pregnancy when I made a home visit. He was soft-spoken and pretty conservative looking, especially compared to Vanessa's busy, swirling, red-haired ball of flower power.

He looked like… Well, he looked like a lawyer. Even though he wore torn jeans, I could easily picture him in court, flipping through pages of arcane legalese on the table before him, focused and alert, waiting for his chance to cross-examine a witness.

"So, Matt, was this pregnancy a surprise to you, too?"

"That's putting it mildly," he said, laughing. "But I think in some ways, it's been easier for me to adjust to the idea than it's been for Vanessa."

"How so?"

"Well, she's been managing everything alone for years – raising her sons, dealing with finances, running the store on Telegraph, just everything. And she's stretched pretty tight, you know? But it's different for me. My life, compared to what it was a couple of years ago, is pretty chill. The stress I was living with when I was a prosecuting attorney is gone, absolutely gone, and I'm feeling more relaxed than I've felt since the day before I started law school."

"Yeah, I can understand that," I said.

"Also, ignorance is bliss. She already has two kids, so she knows what it's like living with a baby in the house. But, me? Not so much. I'm clueless, no idea what I'm in for. So, yeah, it's not what we planned, but I'm pretty okay with it. Looking forward to it, actually," he said, then glanced at Vanessa.

She rolled her eyes. "You're nuts, but you're right about one thing."

"What?"

"You have no clue what you're in for."

Not long after that home visit, Vanessa called me one morning and uttered a single word.

"Damn."

"What?"

"I'm in labor. I'm sure of it. And you're going to tell me I can't have it at home, aren't you?"

I pulled her chart from a stack, flipped it open, glanced at the calendar and said, "Yeah, I'm sorry. It's possible you're more than a month early, Vanessa. I'll come be with you at home until you get active, but then we'll have to go into the hospital."

I didn't have hospital privileges at that time, so I wouldn't be catching her baby once we reached Alta Bates, but I knew Dr. Jackson, my backup doctor, would be kind and permissive. He would manage the birth of Vanessa's baby gently and gracefully.

After calling to alert the doctor that we'd be arriving in a few hours, I drove to the small house in Albany where, indeed, Vanessa was already in good labor. Her boys, ages twelve and fourteen, whom she'd said were "mortally embarrassed at the mere idea of a pregnant mother," had already fled and were staying with friends.

Vanessa labored gracefully, pacing, and cussing now and then that "this whole situation is ridiculous, just fucking ridiculous." Soon it was time to head for the hospital.

As Matt helped her into the car, he turned to me and said, "I thought there'd be more work, more for me to do, but she's really doing fine on her own," and I agreed that, indeed, she was.

Not half an hour after getting settled at the hospital, a thick rope of bloody mucus stained Vanessa's inner thigh, and she began to feel the telltale pressure of a baby's imminent arrival.

Because it was possible the baby was more than a month early, Dr.

Jackson asked if she would permit us to move her to the Delivery Room where there would be more space for a nursery nurse and a neonatologist in the event the baby needed help getting stabilized. Vanessa waved her hand in the air, huffed and grunted a few times, and said, "Just hurry up."

Within a few minutes of getting settled on the birthing bed in the large room, Vanessa gave a huge push, and a head full of hair appeared at the vaginal opening. Even though it was wet, we could all see the obvious.

"It has red hair!" hollered Matt. "Bright red hair! Oh, my God, that's so cool!"

Vanessa, focused and very busy, said, "I don't care if the kid has green or blue hair. Mother of God, just get it out."

With a single push, the head was born, followed immediately by the whole body. A baby girl, with bright red hair and a scrunched up, angry little face. Lusty screams filled the room, and it was quickly apparent the infant wasn't in need of the services of the nursery staff except for bundling her up and keeping her warm.

But...we were looking at a very tiny little baby.

Dr. Jackson and I exchanged glances, and he nodded at me.

While Matt and Vanessa were busy admiring this furious little creature they'd produced, I picked up the fetal stethoscope and listened to Vanessa's belly, which appeared not to have diminished in size at all.

There was another heartbeat.

I nodded to Dr. Jackson, and he touched Vanessa's knee.

"Ma'am?" he said.

No response.

"Uh, ma'am? Ms. Storey? Vanessa?"

Nothing. Where previously Vanessa had had no time to focus on the coming baby, now she had time to focus on nothing *but* the baby.

I touched her cheek and said "Vanessa? Vanessa?"

She struggled to take her eyes off the baby and turned toward me. "What?"

I jerked my head toward the doctor, she looked at him and asked, "What? Is everything okay?"

"Yes, yes. Everything is fine, but..."

"But? What do you mean, *but*? What's wrong?"

"Nothing whatsoever is wrong, but there's another one."

"What are you talking about?"

"There's another one. You're having twins."

Absolute silence.

Matt's jaw dropped open, and Vanessa's big blue eyes grew even bigger.

"Twins? Did you say twins?"

Dr. Jackson nodded.

Then Vanessa did the unexpected. She slammed her knees together and flattened her legs out straight.

And she yelled. "NO. Nonononono *No twins!*"

Oh dear.

"Well…" murmured the doctor, ducking his head to hide a private smile in his beard. "I think you'll…"

"You can't make me!" Vanessa shouted. "You absolutely can *not* make me."

BOOKS BY PEGGY VINCENT

Look out for further books in the
Memoirs of an Urban Midwife series

Also by Peggy Vincent

Baby Catcher: Chronicles of a Modern Midwife, Scribner, 2002
Midwife: A Calling, Ant Press, 2015

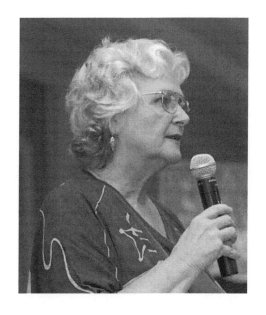

In 1980, after fifteen years as a delivery room nurse, ten years as a childbirth educator, and three years as the director of the first alternative birth center in Berkeley, CA, Peggy Vincent became a Certified Nurse Midwife.

Initially attending only home births, three years later Peggy became the first independent nurse midwife in the area to be granted hospital privileges.

Her memoir, *Baby Catcher: Chronicles of a Modern Midwife*, was published in 2002 by Scribner and has been optioned for a potential TV mini-series.

Midwife: A Calling, was published by Ant Press, in 2015 and heralded Peggy's new series, *Memoirs of an Urban Midwife*. This was followed by *Midwife: A Journey*, Ant Press, 2016. Further books in this series are planned.

Now retired and living in Oakland, CA, with Roger, her husband of more than fifty years, she still enjoys putting in a cameo appearance at special home births now and then.

CONTACT THE AUTHOR, AND LINKS

Email: peggymmv@gmail.com

Facebook: Peggy Vincent

Facebook Book Page: Baby Catcher by Peggy Vincent

Chat with me and other memoir authors and readers in our Facebook group, We Love Memoirs: https://www.facebook.com/groups/welovememoirs/

ACKNOWLEDGEMENTS

My family. They tolerated my weird schedule with grace and understanding.

Our Scandinavian au pairs who cared for my baby when I couldn't be there: Àgi, Mona, and Marianna.

My clients, who handed me their hearts and trusted me with their births.

The women who stood ahead of, beside, and behind me: Rosemary Mann, Judith Flannagan, Carole Hagin, Sandra MacKenzie, Margaret Love, and Bonnie Bruce.

The doctors who provided backup for my midwifery practice: Drs. Jackson, Stallone, Weick, Streitfeld, Kanwit, and Keller.

My editor and Comma Queen, Sally Gambrill in Maine.

My neighbor and Computer Guru, Sally West.

My publisher, Victoria Twead at Ant Press, for doing the things I am incapable of.

ANT PRESS BOOKS

If you enjoyed *Midwife: A Journey*, you may also enjoy these titles:

MEMOIRS

Midwife - A Calling by Peggy Vincent

Chickens, Mules and Two Old Fools by Victoria Twead (Wall Street Journal Top 10 bestseller)

Two Old Fools ~ Olé! by Victoria Twead

Two Old Fools on a Camel by Victoria Twead (thrice New York Times bestseller)

Two Old Fools in Spain Again by Victoria Twead

One Young Fool in Dorset (The Prequel) by VictoriaTwead

One Young Fool in South Africa (The Prequel) by Joe and Victoria Twead

Into Africa with 3 Kids, 13 Crates and a Husband by Ann Patras

More Into Africa with 3 Kids, some Dogs and a Husband by Ann Patras

Fat Dogs and French Estates ~ Part I by Beth Haslam

Fat Dogs and French Estates ~ Part II by Beth Haslam

Fat Dogs and French Estates ~ Part III by Beth Haslam

Simon Ships Out: How One Brave, Stray Cat Became a Worldwide Hero by Jacky Donovan

Smoky: How a Tiny Yorkshire Terrier Became a World War II American Army Hero, Therapy Dog and Hollywood Star by Jacky Donovan

Instant Whips and Dream Toppings: A True-Life Dom Rom Com by Jacky Donovan

Heartprints of Africa: A Family's Story of Faith, Love, Adventure, and Turmoil by Cinda Adams Brooks

How not to be a Soldier: My Antics in the British Army by Lorna

McCann

Moment of Surrender: My Journey Through Prescription Drug Addiction to Hope and Renewal by Pj Laube

Serving is a Pilgrimage by John Basham

FICTION

Parched by Andrew C Branham

A is for Abigail by Victoria Twead (Sixpenny Cross 1)

B is for Bella by Victoria Twead (Sixpenny Cross 2)

CHILDREN'S BOOKS

Seacat Simon: The Little Cat Who Became a Big Hero by Jacky Donovan

The Rise of Agnil by Susan Navas (Agnil's World 1)

Agnil and the Wizard's Orb by Susan Navas (Agnil's World 2)

Agnil and the Tree Spirits by Susan Navas (Agnil's World 3)

Agnil and the Centaur's Secret by Susan Navas (Agnil's World 4)

Morgan and the Martians by Victoria Twead

Chat with the author and other memoir authors and readers at
We Love Memoirs:
https://www.facebook.com/groups/welovememoirs/

18329552R00148

Printed in Great Britain
by Amazon